patrick
HOLFORD

Improve
Your
Digestion

How to make your gut
work for you and
not against you

piatkus

PIATKUS

First published in Great Britain in 1999 by Piatkus Books
This updated and expanded version first published 2017

3 5 7 9 10 8 6 4 2

A CIP catalogue record for this book
is available from the British Library.

ISBN 978-0-349-41400-3

Typeset in Berkeley by M Rules
Printed and bound by CPI Group (UK) Ltd, Croydon, CR0 4YY

Papers used by Piatkus are from well-managed forests
and other responsible sources.

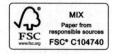

Piatkus
An imprint of
Little, Brown Book Group
Carmelite House
50 Victoria Embankment
London EC4Y 0DZ

An Hachette UK Company
www.hachette.co.uk

www.improvementzone.co.uk

Although the nutrients and dietary changes referred to in this book have been proven safe, those seeking help for specific medical conditions are advised to consult a qualified nutrition therapist, doctor or equivalent health professional. The recommendations given in this book are solely intended as education and information, and should not be taken as medical advice. Neither the author nor the publisher accept liability for readers who choose to self-prescribe.

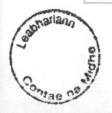

About the Author

Patrick Holford BSc, DipION, FBANT, NTCRP is a leading spokesman on nutrition in the media, specialising in the field of mental health. He is the author of over 30 books, translated into over 20 languages and selling several million copies worldwide, including *The Optimum Nutrition Bible*, *The Low GL-Diet Bible*, *Optimum Nutrition for the Mind* and *Food is Better Medicine than Drugs*.

Patrick started his academic career in the field of psychology. He then became a student of two of the leading pioneers in orthomolecular medicine and psychiatry – the late Dr Carl Pfeiffer and Dr Abram Hoffer. In 1984 he founded the Institute for Optimum Nutrition (ION), an independent educational charity, with his mentor, twice Nobel Prize winner Dr Linus Pauling, as patron. ION has been researching and helping to define what it means to be optimally nourished for the past 32 years and is one of the most respected educational establishments for training nutritional therapists. At ION, Patrick was involved in groundbreaking research showing that multivitamins can increase children's IQ scores – the subject of a *Horizon* documentary in the 1980s. He was one of the first promoters of the importance of zinc, antioxidants, essential fats, low-GL diets and homocysteine-lowering B vitamins and their importance in mental health and Alzheimer's disease prevention.

Patrick is founder of the Food for the Brain Foundation and director of the Brain Bio Centre, the Foundation's treatment centre that specialises in helping those with mental issues ranging from depression to schizophrenia. He is in the Orthomolecular Medicine Hall of Fame and is an honorary fellow of the British Association of Nutritional Therapy, as well as a member of the Nutrition Therapy Council and the Complementary and Natural Healthcare Council. He is also Patron of the South African Association of Nutritional Therapy.

Other books by Patrick Holford

Balance Your Hormones

Boost Your Immune System
(with Jennifer Meek)

Burn Fat Fast (with Kate Staples)

Delicious, Healthy, Sugar-Free
(with Fiona McDonald Joyce)

Food is Better Medicine than
Drugs (with Jerome Burne)

Hidden Food Allergies
(with Dr James Braly)

How to Quit Without Feeling S**t
(with David Miller and Dr
James Braly)

Optimum Nutrition Before,
During and After Pregnancy
(with Susannah Lawson)

Optimum Nutrition for the Mind

Optimum Nutrition for Your
Child (with Deborah Colson)

Optimum Nutrition Made Easy

Say No to Arthritis

Say No to Cancer
(with Liz Efiong)

Say No to Heart Disease

Six Weeks to Superhealth

Smart Food for Smart Kids
(with Fiona McDonald Joyce)

Solve Your Skin Problems
(with Natalie Savona)

Ten Secrets of 100%
Healthy People

Ten Secrets of Healthy Ageing
(with Jerome Burne)

Ten Secrets of 100% Health
Cookbook (with Fiona
McDonald Joyce)

The Alzheimer's Prevention Plan
(with Shane Heaton and
Deborah Colson)

The Chemistry of Connection

The Feel Good Factor

The Homocysteine Solution
(with Dr James Braly)

The 9-day Liver Detox
(with Fiona McDonald Joyce)

The Low-GL Diet Cookbook
(with Fiona McDonald Joyce)

The Low-GL Diet Counter

The Low-GL Diet Bible

The Optimum Nutrition Bible

The Optimum Nutrition
Cookbook (with Judy Ridgway)

The Perfect Pregnancy Cookbook
(with Fiona McDonald Joyce
and Susannah Lawson)

500 Health and Nutrition
Questions Answered

Foreign Editions are listed at
www.patrickholford.com/foreign-editions

Acknowledgements

Many people have helped to research, check and edit this book. My special thanks go to Antony Haynes for his help regarding digestive infections; to Erica White for her expertise and contribution to the section on candidiasis; to Chris Newbold for helping me with the research on probiotics; to Dr Gill Hart for her help researching food intolerances; and to Fiona McDonald Joyce for her delicious gut-friendly recipes. Also thanks to my editor Jan Cutler, and to Jillian Stewart and Tim Whiting at Little, Brown/Piatkus. Most of all thanks to Jo, my manager, and Gaby, my wife, who take care of everything so that I can focus on writing. I would also like to thank all the amazing researchers out there, the unspoken heroes whose studies, collectively, have helped define a whole new, natural, safe and healthy approach to digestive health problems.

Acknowledgements

Contents

Guide to abbreviations
and measures

1 gram (g) = 1,000 milligrams (mg) = 1,000,000 micrograms (mcg or µg)

Most vitamins are measured in milligrams or micrograms. Vitamins A, D and E are also measured in International Units (iu), a measurement designed to standardise the different forms of these vitamins which have different potencies.

1mcg of retinol (mcgRE) = 3.3iu of vitamin A (RE = Retinol Equivalents)

1mcg RE of beta-carotene = 6mcg of beta-carotene

100iu of vitamin D = 2.5mcg

100iu of vitamin E = 67mg

In this book calories means kilocalories (kcals)

References and further
sources of information

Hundreds of references from respected scientific literature have been used in writing this book. Details of specific studies referred to are listed on pages 390–402. On page 385 you will also find a Recommended Reading list, which suggests the best books to read if you wish to dig deeper into the topics covered in this book.

Introduction

The human gut, despite being seen as the somewhat poor relation of the more 'sexy' organs such as the brain and heart, is the hub of good health. Far from being just the 'plumbing' that many people consider it to be, the gut plays numerous vital roles within the body. In fact, good health starts in the gut, because it is here that your inner world (the internal parts of your body) meets the outer world (the food you put into your body). The 'skin' of your digestive tract is wafer thin – a mere one-quarter the thickness of a sheet of paper – but were you to lay it out flat it would cover a surface area of a tennis court ($250m^2$). It is here that all the action happens.

We are frequently told that 'you are what you eat', but contrary to popular belief, you are not. You are what you *can digest and absorb*. Over a lifetime, no less than 100 tonnes of food will pass along the digestive tract, and you'll produce 300,000 litres of digestive juices – 10 litres a day – to break it down. These digestive juices pour into your digestive tract on a mission to break down complex food particles into something simple, such as a sugar, that can be actively transported into your bloodstream and, from there, to all your body's cells.

Amazingly, most of the billions of cells that make up this barrier between your body and the environment are renewed every four days. That is why your digestive system is a hive of activity, only matched by your liver, the central processing organ, and the brain.

Surprising as it may seem, the gut is often considered to be the second brain, because the gut and the brain are in constant communication. Many vital brain-communicating chemicals, such as serotonin, are made in the gut, and this is why having a healthy gut leads to good mental as well as physical health.

Like other animals, we spend our physical lives processing organic matter, extracting nutrients, building materials and fuel, and eliminating the rest. How good we are at this process determines our energy level, longevity, and state of body and mind. A professor at the Harvard School of Medicine once rightly said, 'A strong stomach and a good set of bowels are more important to human happiness than a large amount of brains.'

Before birth, children are connected to their mothers, and they receive nourishment directly into their bloodstream. At birth the umbilical cord is cut and the digestive system takes over. As we take over our own nourishment we lose that direct maternal dependence, and become totally dependent on external sources of food. Our very survival depends on it.

At one time we depended upon our senses of sight, touch, taste and smell to guide us towards nourishment in the natural world. Nowadays, however, our senses, cleverly manipulated by artificially coloured, flavour-enhanced and sweetened convenience foods, have become our masters. We have, for example, a need for essential fats. In our mouths, accordingly, are fat receptors that respond to the ingestion of essential fats. If, on the other hand, we eat fake fats designed to simulate the texture of fat, the fat receptors are not so strongly stimulated and do not pass on the message of satisfaction. Consequently, we continue to crave fat and continue to choose the wrong kind of fat, causing ourselves many long-term health problems.

Our food, and the urban world we inhabit, has denatured us. We no longer receive the correct bacterial exposure in our over-sanitised world, and, consequently, the fingerprint of our gut bacteria has altered to the point where many people become increasingly intolerant, or even allergic to various foods.

Plants exist to capture energy from the sun and convert it into sugars that feed, via their roots, microorganisms that make up the soil. Modern farming methods destroy the careful balance of the soil, and thus the health of the plants, which we then eat.

Similarly, our food and the bacteria in our guts are like the soil of our system. Our 'roots' are the villi, the protrusions from the gut wall that feed off what we eat. We 'gather' food to feed these bacteria, but modern food is destroying this careful balance between the body and its bacteria, between humans and microorganisms in the gut.

The role of gut bacteria in health has come a long way since I started studying nutrition, and the evidence for their benefit has grown exponentially since I wrote the first version of this book back in 1998. I remember when scientists first identified the 'human' strains of bacteria and cultivated them to promote gut health, reported in a damning newspaper article headed 'Let them eat shit'. Yet, so much scientific evidence now highlights the importance of the right balance of bacteria in the gut, not only for good health but also for weight loss.

Taking in all the nutrients we need at optimal amounts is not only a recipe for a long and healthy physical life, but it also helps us to achieve our full potential as human beings. Because the body knows when it is receiving everything it requires for its survival, our energy and consciousness can be directed towards fulfilling other needs.

The consequences of sub-optimum nutrition are evident in the increasing incidence of digestive problems and diseases. Every other person, it seems, suffers from bloating, indigestion or irritable bowel syndrome (IBS), a food intolerance or an allergy. Most are constipated, and colorectal cancer is fast becoming the number-one killer of people under the age of 50.

There is no doubt that many of us are digging our own graves with a knife and fork. No longer is most of society's suffering the result of poverty. Indeed, much of the Western world's illness is the consequence of eating too much, rather than too little, and eating the wrong kinds of food.

As a result, there is a quiet epidemic of digestive problems, including indigestion, infections, acid reflux, IBS, stomach bugs, ulcers, Crohn's disease, colitis and diverticulitis, candidiasis and consequent chronic fatigue.

Whether or not you are currently suffering from any of these ailments, the chances are that you could tune up your digestion and reap rewards in terms of extra health and energy. This book is designed to help you do just that.

Parts I and II explain the digestive system, describing each step along the way, from the beginnings of digesting your food to the act of absorbing nutrients into the body. I explain what goes wrong and how you can adjust your eating to ensure optimal digestion and absorption, which foods to avoid and which to eat more of.

Part III focuses on specific digestive problems – from indigestion to stomach ulcers, and heartburn to IBS and bloating – and the solutions that can help to restore your digestive health. If you have developed a gut infection, be it candida, dysbiosis or a less common gut infection, I'll show you how to restore your gut health. I also focus on inflammatory bowel disorders, from Crohn's to ulcerative colitis.

Part IV puts it all together into an action plan that you can use to clean up your digestion, detoxify your body and experience the consistent energy and clarity of mind that come from optimally nourishing yourself.

Part V gives you delicious digestion-friendly recipes, to help you enjoy the process of becoming, and staying, digestively healthy.

In each chapter you will find simple guidelines for you to follow to improve your digestion. With current testing methods and recent advances in natural treatments, the vast majority of digestive problems can be solved with relative ease, little expense and no need for invasive tests or treatment. The digestive tract is one of the most regenerative parts of the body and, with the most suitable diet, the majority of digestive problems can be swiftly resolved. For those without any apparent digestive problems, following the guidelines in this book may improve your ability to derive energy from food, thus increasing your vitality and resistance to disease.

I wish you the very best of health,

Patrick Holford

PART I

IMPROVING YOUR DIGESTION

CHAPTER 1

The Digestive System – the Very Beginning

The gut is as vital to our health as our heart, yet few people know much about the workings of this amazing organ. This chapter will begin to address that. The digestive tract, which is technically known as the gastrointestinal tract, is about 10m long and has various organs attached to it which produce digestive juices.

Although it is inside the body, the digestive tract is in contact with the outside world, because it is here that food is broken down from the larger pieces that we eat into smaller particles that can then be absorbed into the body.

The stages of digestion

Surprising as it may seem, digestion starts as soon as you think about, smell or see food you want to eat because it is at this point that your body starts producing digestion enzymes in anticipation of what is to come.

The mouth

The first act of digestion starts in the mouth, where the act of chewing food begins to physically break it down. Leading into the mouth are salivary glands, which, unsurprisingly, produce saliva. Saliva has a dual role: it lubricates the food to make it easy to swallow and it begins to break it down, due to the action of the digestive enzyme ptyalin. Food then passes down the throat, along the oesophagus and into the stomach.

The stomach

The stomach is a carefully controlled environment with a seal at the top (the cardiac sphincter) and at the bottom (the pyloric sphincter) to prevent the acidic digestive juices from escaping. About 2 litres of these juices are produced each day by cells in the stomach wall. They help to further digest food, especially protein, and to kill off bacteria and other undesirable microorganisms. They also help to prepare vitamin B_{12} for absorption. The food, which by this stage is known as chyme, can be present in the stomach for two to five hours before it is released into the small intestine.

The small intestine

Broadly speaking, the small intestine is where absorption of nutrients takes place, but this doesn't happen immediately. The first part of the small intestine – the duodenum – is the hotspot of digestion, because it is here that digestive juices from the liver and pancreas pour in via the bile duct and the pancreatic duct. As you will learn later in the chapter, these are the main players in further breaking down food, although the wall of the small intestine also produces its own digestive juices.

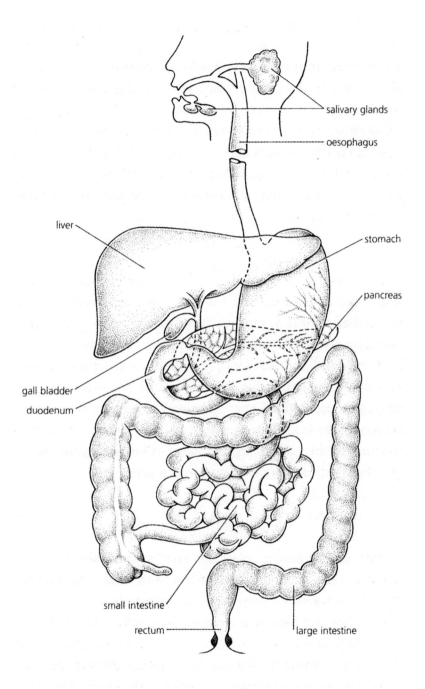

The digestive system

After the duodenum is the middle section of the small intestine – the jejunum – and it is here that most nutrients are absorbed into the body. The last part of the small intestine, called the ileum, is connected to the large intestine, or colon.

The chyme is further digested, more nutrients are absorbed, and what is left is passed along the small intestine by a wave-like muscular action called peristalsis. Billions of bacteria live in the small intestine, forming our first line of immune defence against infections and keeping the gut healthy.

The large intestine (colon)

Whereas the small intestine is primarily involved in digestion and absorption, the large intestine prepares what is left (mainly undigested fibres, unabsorbed food, bacteria and dead cells) for elimination. These two areas – the 'kitchen' area (small intestine) and the 'waste' area (large intestine) – are kept separate by a muscular seal called the ileo-caecal valve. If this valve doesn't work properly, there is a danger that undesirable organisms will move from the large intestine into the small intestine, leading to intestinal infections (see pages 210–222).

Although some nutrients are absorbed from the colon, its main role is to reabsorb water from the chyme and pass waste material along, ready for elimination. About a litre of water a day is reabsorbed in this way. Again, peristaltic muscle contractions help to move material along into the rectum, the last part of the colon. When this is full, it triggers defecation.

As well as eliminating unabsorbed food matter, defecation also removes other substances from the body, including dead blood cells and excess cholesterol.

Tackling digestive problems

With such a complex system it's little wonder that digestive problems can be so tricky to tackle. However, they are best considered by asking three fundamental questions: (i) Are you digesting your food properly? (ii) Are you absorbing properly? and (iii) Are you eliminating properly?

Before we move on, it's important to note that these three stages – digestion, absorption and elimination – don't just apply to physical material. After all, isn't this what we do with psychological material too? When you read a newspaper, for example, you 'digest' certain stories, absorb some facts or ideas, then eliminate the rest. Quite often, people who have physical problems with elimination also find it difficult to let go of things, both physically and mentally. They may hoard unnecessary psychological baggage. We will explore the link between psychological 'digestion' and physical digestion in Chapter 11 – Do You Have the Guts to be Happy and Stress-Free?

When tuning up your digestion, it's best to work from the top down. For this reason the next section looks at the first key process – chewing – followed by digestion and the role of digestive enzymes.

It's good to chew

As simple as it might sound, the act of digesting and absorbing nutrients from food is a highly complex and carefully orchestrated affair. As soon as you think about food, see it, smell it and taste it, the digestive tract starts preparing the right digestive juices to deal with the meal.

The body produces about 10 litres of digestive juices every day, but how does it know how much to produce? If you eat protein rather than carbohydrate, or a large meal rather than a small meal, the amount and type of digestive juices needed will be very different. Also, how does the body know if a food is good or bad for you? Your body is preparing for these different aspects of digestion even before you swallow a piece of food.

Firstly, your eyes recognise what is edible and attractive, but your nose is actually more important because smell involves taking in tiny particles of the food. If a food has gone bad, it might not always look bad, but it will certainly smell bad. That's why no animal ever eats a piece of food without smelling it first. As food enters your mouth, the nature of the food is being analysed, and this triggers the production and release of different digestive enzymes. This process is helped by smelling and chewing your food. This explains why wolfing your food down without chewing it properly first can give you indigestion.

The stomach, the first major stop along the way to complete digestion, doesn't have teeth. That is why it is critical to chew your food well before you swallow it. Some people say you should chew each mouthful 30 times. That may be a bit excessive, but it makes the point. For some people who have compromised digestion this can make a big difference. Chewing does much more than just signal to your digestion what's to come. As I pointed out earlier, the salivary glands in the mouth release large amounts of saliva, which contains the digestive enzyme ptyalin. Ptyalin helps to break down large carbohydrate particles into smaller ones (which is why, if you keep chewing a piece of bread, it will actually get digested in your mouth). So, the more you chew, the better you prepare your food by pre-digesting it, and the less work your digestive system has to do. Obviously, chewing also physically breaks down food into smaller pieces, increasing the surface area of your food and making it easier for the digestive juices to do their work.

Gut reactions

The digestive system does much more than digest food. Scientists are discovering that the digestive system 'thinks' and 'feels' and might act almost as a second brain. Early models of the brain and cognition proposed that what we call thinking and feeling boiled down to the sending and receiving of chemical messengers called neurotransmitters and hormones. Now scientists are discovering that there is a vast amount of neurotransmitter and hormone activity in the digestive tract. Serotonin, the 'happy' neurotransmitter, is largely produced in the gut (see Chapter 11 for more on this). In addition to this, there are more immune cells in the gut than there are in the rest of the body. These three – neurotransmitters, hormones and immune cells – are the chemicals of communication of what is known as the neuro-endo-immune system, or to put it simply, the intelligence of the body. It is this highly sophisticated network that allows us to keep responding appropriately to our ever-changing environment.

In practical terms, this means that you can't separate thoughts, feelings and physical reactions. What you eat, what you think and feel about what you eat, and what you think and feel about when you eat, all have a bearing on the end result. This is why, for optimum nourishment, it is good to choose the most nutritious foods, prepare them in a way that you like, eat the food consciously, and have good thoughts as you are actually eating.

This is the complete opposite of the way many people eat today. Often, when I ask clients what they have eaten in the last two days, they struggle to remember. Lunch was something grabbed from a sandwich shop and eaten unconsciously, amid stressful thoughts and feelings. Much of our food is eaten on the run. How different this is from the culture of Mediterranean countries, for example, where everyone helps to prepare the food, and to set the table, while family and friends take time to enjoy the feast.

No wonder they have fewer heart attacks!

Summary – Chapter 1

Next time you eat a meal:

- Select high-quality foods and prepare them so that they look and taste good.
- Smell your food before you eat it.
- Think about its origin and that these molecules of food will literally become you.
- Chew each mouthful completely before beginning the next.
- Take some time away from your busy life for your meals, whether you are eating alone or in good company.

CHAPTER 2

Enzymes –
the Keys of Life

The food we eat is made of large, complex molecules that can't possibly be used within our bodies. As we have seen, they first have to be broken down into much smaller particles that are not only physically able to get through the wall of the digestive tract but are also beneficial to the body. This breaking down process is the job of digestive enzymes.

Digestive enzymes are produced in large amounts at different stages along the digestive tract. If you don't produce enough of them to digest your food efficiently, you can get indigestion, bloating and flatulence. The long-term effects of having undigested food in your system, however, are more insidious and can lead to a greater risk of conditions such as inflammatory bowel syndrome, digestive infections (such as candidiasis), food intolerances and even cancer.

Let's look at the very important – if somewhat complex – process of breaking down food.

Digesting carbohydrate

Carbohydrate digestion begins in the mouth, through the action of the enzyme ptyalin. As we have seen, ptyalin is an amylase (an enzyme that digests carbohydrate). Carbohydrate is not further digested in the stomach, so it can theoretically pass straight into the duodenum (the first part of the small intestine). Special cells in the pancreas then produce large amounts of amylase enzymes that pour out of the pancreatic duct into the duodenum, ready to break down the carbohydrate. The pancreas also produces alkaline substances that help to neutralise the acid that was mixed into the food while it was in the stomach. Amylase enzymes break down complex sugar molecules called polysaccharides (for example, in grains) into simpler sugars such as malt (the sugar that can be produced from grains such as wheat or barley); however, the process is not yet over for carbohydrates. More amylase enzymes are produced in cells that line the upper part of the small intestine; these can break down sugars such as maltose (known as a disaccharide) into the simplest kinds of sugar, called monosaccharides. The most important monosaccharide is glucose – this is fuel for the human body and the ultimate goal of carbohydrate digestion.

Evolutionarily speaking, around a million years ago we appear to have developed the DNA (our body's instructions) for making all kinds of different amylases, and this coincided with the time that our ancestors discovered fire and started cooking foods. Cooking, much like digestion, helped to make more carbohydrates from nature available to us with less digestive effort. Cooking also made meat easier to digest. As a consequence our gut length shortened and this also paralleled a growth in brain size.[1]

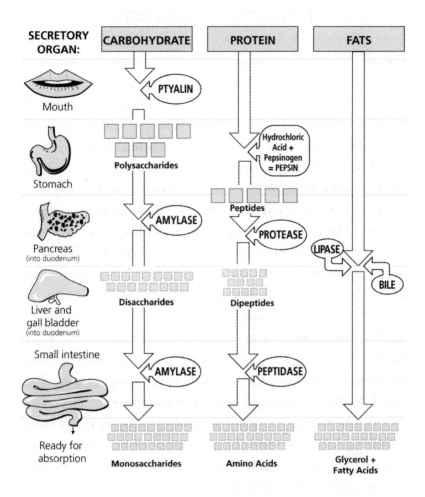

Digestive enzymes

Digesting protein

In contrast to carbohydrate, protein is digested principally in the stomach. For this reason the stomach produces two substances: hydrochloric acid and an enzyme called pepsinogen. Hydrochloric acid (commonly called stomach acid) gets to work on the big protein molecules straight away, but its action alone is limited. When the body combines pepsinogen and hydrochloric acid, however, a very powerful enzyme called pepsin is created. This starts to break down complex proteins into relatively small chunks of amino acids, called peptides. These peptides are further broken down into individual amino acids by more protein-digesting enzymes (collectively known as proteases) which enter the duodenum from the pancreas.

Protein digestion is also done by protease enzymes produced by special cells in the first part of the small intestine. The end result, if all goes well, is that complex proteins become simple amino acids, ready for absorption.

Digesting fat

Protein and carbohydrate are effectively water soluble and can therefore be acted on by the enzymes in digestive juices. Fat, however, repels water and is thus impervious to these enzymes. For this reason, the first stage of digesting fat, called emulsification, prepares the fat particles for digestion. This is done by a substance called bile, which is made in the liver and stored in the gall bladder. Bile breaks down large fat globules into tiny droplets of fat. The result of this, which could be compared to turning a football into 15 tennis balls – is that a much greater surface area of the fat is exposed to the digestive juices. Once again, the pancreas plays a key role, because the digestive juices it produces and sends into the duodenum contain lipase, a fat-digesting enzyme.

Bile then enters the duodenum along the bile duct and starts to break the fat down into tiny particles. Meanwhile, lipase also enters the duodenum and actually digests the fat ready for absorption.

Bile is produced by the liver and concentrated in the gallbladder and is a combination of alkaline salts, which help to neutralise stomach acid; lecithin, the primary emulsifying factor; and cholesterol. Whenever you eat fat, the body gets ready by squeezing the gall bladder to secrete bile into the digestive tract.

What causes indigestion?

One of the main reasons for indigestion is the body not producing enough of all the enzymes I've just described, with the result that it cannot digest food properly. This means that incompletely digested food hangs around in the small intestine feeding the bacteria that live there. These bacteria produce gas, resulting in bloating, flatulence and digestive pain. The release of stomach acid can also be a problem (see Chapter 4). If the body has particular difficulty digesting fat, the stools tend to be very buoyant and light in colour. Also, since the goodness in the food isn't getting into the body, instead of feeling better after a meal the person affected often feels worse.

The body cells, such as those in the pancreas, depend on vitamins and minerals to produce enzymes. But if you're not digesting your food you don't get the nutrients you need to make these enzymes – and so it's a vicious circle. Nowadays, it is relatively easy to find out if a person isn't digesting properly, using two non-invasive tests. The first, known as the Gastrogram, was invented by Dr John McLaren Howard at Biolab in London (see Resources). It involves swallowing special capsules that transmit messages showing the efficiency of stomach acid secretion, the speed at which the stomach is emptying into the small intestine, and the efficiency of pancreatic enzymes. The other method is stool analysis (see Resources).

If the stool contains undigested protein, fats or carbohydrates, this can also identify a digestion problem. This method is more commonly used and has replaced the Gastrogram.

The first action to take if you have indigestion is to supplement with digestive enzymes, the main three being amylase, protease and lipase. Digestive enzymes come in many different forms, ranging from natural compounds (which will be rich in one or other enzyme) to combinations of amylase, protease and lipase. If, having supplemented digestive enzymes with your meal, you feel instantly better afterwards, that's a good sign that indigestion is your problem. Foods that are rich in digestive enzymes include papaya and pineapple. On page 327 I explain more about digestive enzymes taken as supplements.

Some digestive enzymes also contain lactase, which is the enzyme for digesting lactose, the primary sugar in milk. Others contain an additional enzyme called alpha-galactosidase. This enzyme aids digestion of some of the naturally indigestible compounds found in certain vegetables and beans, hence preventing wind.

Here are the common ingredients you might find in a digestive enzyme supplement:

	Digests Fat	Digests Protein	Digests Carbohydrate
Papain (from papaya)		✔	
Bromelain (from pineapple)	✔	✔	
Pancreatin (extract of pancreas)	✔	✔	✔
Ox bile extract	✔		
Amylase			✔
Protease		✔	
Lipase	✔		

Another key ingredient in digestive enzyme supplements is betaine hydrochloride (betaine HCl), which is stomach acid. Whether or not you need a supplement containing this is discussed fully in Chapter 4. Some supplements also contain amylo-glucosidase (also called glucoamylase), which helps to digest glucosides found in cruciferous vegetables such as cabbage, kale, cauliflower, broccoli and Brussels sprouts, thereby reducing wind. There's also an enzyme called invertase, which breaks down sugar into glucose.

If you're vegetarian, it's best to choose a digestive enzyme supplement that provides amylase, protease and lipase. If you're not, pancreatin is a safe bet. You can test the effects of these enzyme supplements by crushing them and stirring them into a thick porridge. If the product is good, the porridge will become liquid in 30 minutes.

Although there is no harm in taking digestive enzymes on an ongoing basis, correcting digestive enzyme levels with supplements paves the way for increasing body levels of nutrients. Once this is achieved, digestion often improves of its own accord and then the digestive enzyme supplements might no longer be necessary. For this reason I'd recommend taking a digestive enzyme supplement with each main meal for a month, then stopping. If lack of enzymes is a problem you should start to feel relief in a day or two. The best digestive enzymes contain all the enzymes mentioned above.

Enzyme-friendly foods

Problems with digestion aren't just about a lack of digestive enzymes. If you overeat, this is going to strain your body's ability to digest even under the best of circumstances. Grazing rather than gorging – eating little and often – is therefore a great help to digestion. So too is eating raw foods, because they contain significant amounts of enzymes.

Helsinki biochemist and Nobel Prize winner Professor Artturi Virtanen showed that enzymes in uncooked foods are released in the mouth when vegetables are chewed. When these foods are crushed, the enzymes come into contact with the food and start the act of digestion.

These food enzymes are not denatured by stomach acid, as some researchers have suggested, but in fact remain active throughout the digestive tract. Extensive tests by Kaspar Tropp in Wurzburg have shown that the human body has a way of protecting enzymes that pass through the gut so that more than half reach the colon intact. There they alter the intestinal flora by binding free oxygen, reducing the chances of fermentation and putrefaction in the intestines (a factor linked to cancer of the colon). In so doing they also help to create conditions in which lactic-acid-forming beneficial bacteria can grow.

Some foods do contain enzyme blockers; for example, lentils, beans and chickpeas contain trypsin-inhibitors (which prevent protein from complete digestion), which is why they can produce a lot of gas. This anti-enzyme factor is destroyed, however, by sprouting the food or by cooking it.

The two main digestive enzymes, amylase and protease, are found in many foods. For centuries, humans have utilised these food enzymes in order to make fermented foods, which means that the food is effectively 'pre-digested' before we eat it. Yoghurt and sauerkraut are examples of fermented foods. As we have seen above, however, raw foods also contain these enzymes. They become active when we chew but are destroyed by cooking, highlighting the value of eating fruit and vegetables raw. These foods, therefore, need to be chewed properly to liberate and activate the enzymes they contain.

Enzymes naturally present in raw foods

Food	Digests: Enzyme:	Sugars Amylase	Protein Protease	Fat Lipase	Free radicals Peroxidase Catalase
Apple					✔
Banana		✔			
Cabbage		✔			
Corn		✔			
Egg (raw)		✔	✔	✔	✔
Grapes					✔
Honey (raw)		✔			✔
Kidney beans		✔	✔		
Mango					✔
Milk (raw)		✔			✔
Mushroom		✔	✔		✔
Pineapple		✔	✔		
Rice		✔			
Soya beans			✔		
Sweet potato		✔			
Wheat		✔	✔		

The chart above shows those foods that have been found to contain significant levels of health-promoting enzymes. This list, however, is far from complete, as many foods have not been investigated. Suffice to say that raw fruit and vegetables make a major contribution to our ability to digest, absorb and be nourished by our food.

Summary – Chapter 2

You can improve your ability to digest food by following these enzyme-friendly steps:

- Take a digestive-enzyme supplement with each main meal (see Chapter 31 for more on this).
- Avoid overeating. Eat little and often.
- Eat as much raw food as possible, chewing it well.
- Choose enzyme-friendly foods, such as papaya, pineapple, sprouted beans and seeds, and fermented foods such as yoghurt.

CHAPTER 3

Food Combining – Facts and Fiction

Many people find that certain types or combinations of foods don't suit them. Based on this observation and his research into health and nutrition in the 1930s, Dr Howard Hay devised a diet plan, popularly known as 'food combining', which has helped millions of people towards better health. The key suggestions in Dr Hay's original theory were to eat 'alkaline-forming' foods, avoid refined and heavily processed foods, eat fruit on its own, and to avoid combining protein-rich and carbohydrate-rich foods in the same meal or snack.

Eating alkaline-forming foods, by the way, means eating less protein, especially animal protein, rich in amino acids. Alkaline foods, such as fruits and vegetables, are high in the alkalising minerals potassium and magnesium, as well as calcium and sodium.

As we have seen, protein and carbohydrate are digested differently. Carbohydrate digestion begins in the mouth when the digestive enzyme amylase, which is in the saliva, starts to interact with the food you chew. Once you swallow food and it

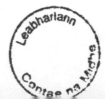

enters the relatively acid environment of the stomach, amylase stops working. Only when the food leaves the stomach, where the digestive environment becomes more alkaline, can the next wave of amylase enzymes (this time secreted into the small intestine from the pancreas) complete the digestion of carbohydrate.

Protein, on the other hand, is not digested at all in the mouth. It needs the acid environment of the stomach and may remain there for several hours until all the complex proteins are broken down into small groups of amino acids. The common, overly simplistic, approach to food combining is therefore to separate carbohydrate and protein foods because they are digested differently.

A food-combining myth?

Of course, since foods aren't exclusively either carbohydrate or protein, in practical terms separating protein and carbohydrate actually means not combining *concentrated* protein foods with *concentrated* starch foods. Meat is 50 per cent protein/0 per cent carbohydrate; potatoes are 8 per cent protein/90 per cent carbohydrate. In between are beans, lentils, rice, wheat and quinoa.

Beans means . . .

Beans contain both protein and carbohydrate, and this is often given as the reason why certain kinds of beans produce flatulence. It is now known, however, that this is not the reason for beans' boisterous reputation. In some beans there are proteins, such as lectins, which cannot be easily digested by the enzymes in our small intestine, so these undigested food particles then feed bacteria that are lower down the gut, creating gas. When you eat beans, you not only feed yourself but you also feed these bacteria. These bacteria produce gas after a good meal of lectin – hence the flatulence. It's got nothing to do with food combining. Many healthy cultures throughout the world have evolved to eat a diet in which beans or lentils are a staple food without suffering from digestive problems.

So where exactly do we draw the line when it comes to protein and carbohydrate content, if we draw a line at all? A brief excursion into our primitive past might solve the puzzle.

The evolution of human digestion

The general consensus is that we, the human race, have been eating a predominantly vegetarian diet for millions of years, with the occasional helping of meat or fish. Unlike mammals that have a ruminant-like digestive tract and slowly digest even the most indigestible fibrous foods (for example, cows), we have a much speedier and technologically advanced digestive system that produces a whole series of different enzyme secretions. And, unlike our ancestors, the apes, we have a longer small intestine, better for fully digesting our more carefully selected food, and a shorter large intestine, because we no longer constantly eat a ton of fibrous foods. The system is more efficient but can only handle foods that are easier to digest – fruit, young leaves and certain vegetables (no tough stalks for us!). Evolutionary theorists believe this 'latest model' digestive system did two things: first, it gave us the motivation to improve our mental and sensory processing so we would know when and where to find the food we needed; and second, it gave us the nutrients to develop a more advanced brain and nervous system.

Did early humans eat meat and two veg?

I suggest we have three basic ways of digesting food. The first is for digesting concentrated protein (meat, fish and eggs). To digest these foods we have to produce vast amounts of stomach acid and protein-digesting enzymes. When our early hunter-gatherer ancestors hunted down and killed an animal, they would probably have eaten their catch, organs and all, as fast as possible before it went off and other predators moved in. They would therefore often have days eating mostly concentrated animal protein, with perhaps just a peppering of carbohydrate vegetables thrown in to bulk out the rations. I doubt they were concerned about adding in enough to constitute what we think of as a 'balanced' meal!

Fruit – the lone ranger

As fruit is seasonal, at certain times of the year early humans would have had access to various fruits, and since fruit is basically the best fuel for instant energy, requiring very little digestion, we are good at producing the enzymes and hormones necessary to process its simple carbohydrates. My guess is that we mainly ate fruit on its own. After all, once you've chomped your way through three bananas, you have little motivation to go digging up vegetables.

Also, many kinds of soft fruit ferment rapidly once they're ripe. They'll do the same if you put them in a warm, acidic

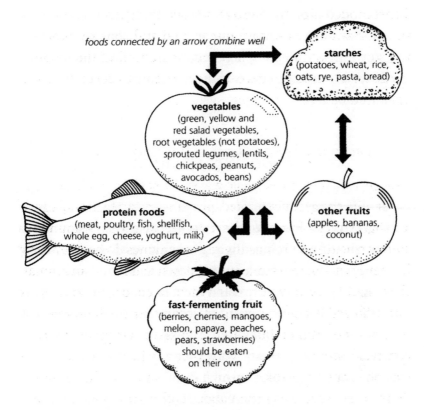

foods connected by an arrow combine well

starches
(potatoes, wheat, rice, oats, rye, pasta, bread)

vegetables
(green, yellow and red salad vegetables, root vegetables (not potatoes), sprouted legumes, lentils, chickpeas, peanuts, avocados, beans)

protein foods
(meat, poultry, fish, shellfish, whole egg, cheese, yoghurt, milk)

other fruits
(apples, bananas, coconut)

fast-fermenting fruit
(berries, cherries, mangoes, melon, papaya, peaches, pears, strawberries) should be eaten on their own

Food combinations – dos and don'ts

environment, which is what the stomach is. And this is what happens if you eat steak and some melon in close succession. Although eating fermented foods is good for the gut, foods that ferment while *in* the gut present a problem, because fermented foods are really pre-digested foods, whereas eating food that ferments inside you creates gas.

Dr Hay's advice to eat fruit separately makes a lot of sense because fruit takes about 30 minutes to pass through the stomach, whereas concentrated protein takes two to three hours. This means that the best time to eat fruit as a snack is more than 30 minutes before a meal or not less than one to two hours after a meal, or possibly more if you eat a lot of concentrated protein. The only exception to this is combining fruits that don't readily ferment – such as bananas, apples and coconut – with complex carbohydrate-rich foods such as oats. Apple porridge, or a whole rye banana sandwich, would therefore be fine.

A healthy balance

Most of the time, our earliest ancestors in Africa seem to have eaten a largely varied vegan diet, with occasional meat or fish (although things changed when we migrated out of Africa): that means leaf vegetables, root vegetables, nuts and seeds. This, I propose, is the third and most common food grouping that our digestion is designed to accommodate – a mixture of foods containing carbohydrate and protein (though nothing as protein-dense as meat). I don't see any problem in combining rice, lentils, beans, vegetables, nuts and seeds.

Although separating concentrated protein from concentrated carbohydrate might make digestion a little easier, it is now known that adding protein to a carbohydrate meal slows down the release of the sugars contained in carbohydrate, making it easier to keep your blood sugar level stable. This is particularly helpful as part of a weight-loss strategy and for keeping energy levels even. Protein and carbohydrate separation might therefore be very beneficial for restoring proper digestion in those with enzyme deficiency, but is not necessarily a rule for life and is not a good idea if you want to lose weight.

If you have tried a food-combining – or more correctly a non-combining – strategy and still have digestion problems, you might have a digestive-enzyme deficiency, a food intolerance or dysbiosis, all of which will be discussed in detail in this book.

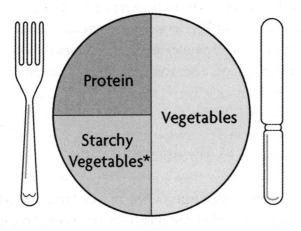

Combining foods in a meal

* The types of starchy vegetables we should be eating include butternut squash, parsnip and beetroot. These are known as 'low-GL' vegetables, and I explain about these in the box on page 53.

Summary – Chapter 3

In general, to give your digestion a helping hand:

- Eat 80 per cent alkaline-forming foods and 20 per cent acid-forming foods. This means eating large quantities of vegetables, fruit and protein foods such as beans, lentils and whole grains, and lesser quantities of meat, fish, cheese and eggs.
- Eat fast-fermenting and acid fruits on their own as snacks. Most soft fruits ferment quickly. These include peaches, plums, mangoes, strawberries and melons. Highly acid fruits (although alkaline-forming) might also inhibit the digestion of

carbohydrate. This includes oranges, lemons, grapefruit and pineapple. All these fruits require little digestion, releasing their natural fructose content quickly. Eat them on their own as a snack.

- Eat animal protein on its own or with vegetables.
- Concentrated proteins – such as meat, fish, hard cheese and eggs – require large amounts of stomach acid and about three hours to be digested. Don't combine fast-releasing foods, or food that ferments, with animal protein. Either have with just vegetables, or with a small portion of 'slow-releasing' carbohydrates; for example, have half a plate of vegetables, one-quarter of the plate as protein and one-quarter as low-GL starchy carbohydrate.
- Avoid all refined carbohydrates such as white pasta, rice and bread. Eat unrefined, slow-releasing carbohydrates such as brown basmati rice, and whole grains such as oats, barley, rye and ancient but not modern wheat (see Chapter 9 for more on this). Fast-releasing fruits that don't readily ferment, such as bananas, apples and coconut, can be combined with slow-releasing carbohydrate cereals such as oats and millet.
- In the mornings, don't eat until your body is fully awake. Leave at least an hour between waking and eating. If you exercise in the morning, eat afterwards. Never start your day with a stimulant (tea, coffee or a cigarette) because the 'stress' state created by this inhibits digestion. If you do take a stimulant, leave an hour between it and your breakfast.

CHAPTER 4

Passing the Acid Test

S tomach acid (hydrochloric acid) is not an enzyme but it is one of the most critical factors in digestion. Too much or too little are common causes of digestive problems. Not only is stomach acid required for all protein digestion, but it is also necessary for mineral absorption, and it is your body's first line of defence against infections, effectively sterilising your food. Stomach secretions, called 'intrinsic factor', are also vital for the absorption of vitamin B_{12}. A lack of stomach acid leaves you unable to digest properly and thereby prone to gut infections, which disturb your healthy balance of gut bacteria, a condition known as dysbiosis. This can lead to indigestion, particularly after high-protein meals, and the risk of developing food allergies and intolerances because undigested large protein molecules are more likely to stimulate immune reactions in the small intestine. Also, all this undigested food feeds the bacteria in the gut, creating gas. This is particularly a problem if you have an overgrowth of the wrong kind of gut bacteria (see Chapter 7 for more on this).

One of the most common reasons for a lack of stomach acid is zinc deficiency, because the production of hydrochloric acid is dependent on a sufficient intake of zinc. Hydrochloric acid production often declines in old age, as does zinc status. About a third of people aged over 60 have low stomach acid, and 40 per cent of women over 80 produce no stomach acid at all. Stomach acid secretion declines by about 20 per cent per decade from the age of 30. The average 20-something-year-old produces 150mg per hour, whereas the average 60-something-year-old produces 50mg per hour.

The symptoms of low stomach acid include burping after eating; bad breath; indigestion, especially associated with protein-rich foods; upper abdominal pain; flatulence; bloating; diarrhoea or constipation. Another indicator is feeling full shortly after eating, or the sensation that food is slow to pass from the stomach. Another is heartburn due to belching, which lets some stomach acid into the oesophagus. This is called gastro-esophageal reflux disorder or GERD (see Chapter 17 for solutions for GERD, acid reflux and indigestion).

Stress also suppresses the production of stomach acid. This is because when we are stressed the body channels energy towards the 'fight' or 'flight' response and away from digestion, so eating when you're stressed, or on the move, is definitely a bad idea.

The nutritional solution to the problem of too little stomach acid is to take a digestive enzyme supplement containing betaine hydrochloride, plus at least 15mg of zinc in an easily absorbable form such as zinc citrate. But you have to be a little careful – if you unknowingly had a stomach ulcer, this could make you feel worse (see Chapter 17 for more details).

Overacidity

Some people produce too much stomach acid, in which case supplementing betaine hydrochloride is likely to make matters worse rather than better. In most cases overacidity indicates that a person's stomach is having a hard time. When a baby eats something unsuitable, the baby quickly vomits or gets diarrhoea. Continual dietary abuse hardens the stomach to such an immediate response but inflames and aggravates the stomach wall.

Alcohol, coffee, tea and aspirin all irritate the gut wall, as does an excessive intake of wheat products. Very hot drinks and spicy foods, especially chilli, are also stomach-unfriendly.

Meat, fish, eggs and other concentrated proteins stimulate acid production. And this can aggravate the situation further because stomach acid will irritate an unhealthy and inflamed stomach lining that, when healthy, would produce its own protective mucus secretions. The conventional medical approach is to suppress the inflammation by giving a drug such as Tagamet (cimetidine); however, this doesn't deal with the underlying cause, which is eating and drinking the wrong foods. Underacidity is far more common than overacidity.

Stomach ulcers

The result of having a stomach-unfriendly diet is often stomach ulcers. Actually, there are two kinds of ulcer: peptic ulcers, which are located in the stomach; and duodenal ulcers, which are located just after the stomach in the duodenum. The simplistic view is that ulcers are due to excess stomach acid, but in fact the body is well designed to protect itself from its own healthy digestive juices. The trouble is that eating and drinking the wrong things damages the digestive tract, which is then further aggravated by stomach acid. Cutting back on irritant foods and high-protein foods certainly helps reduce the immediate aggravation of existing ulcers, but the ulcers still need to be healed.

Vitamin A is especially important for healing ulcers, whereas omega-3 fats (found in fish oils) help to calm inflammation. Vitamin C (ascorbic acid), while helpful for healing ulcers, is a weak acid and can therefore make matters worse. In fact, if you supplement vitamin C and experience fairly rapid gastric pain or burning, it is well worth asking your doctor to check whether or not you have the early stages of an ulcer.

Instead, supplement calcium or magnesium ascorbate (which are alkaline forms of vitamin C). Furthermore, the minerals calcium and magnesium are particularly alkaline and tend to have a calming effect on those suffering from excess acidity.

The helicobacter story

The majority of people who have ulcers have been found to be infected with a bacteria called *Helicobacter pylori* which, unlike other bacteria, can survive in the acid environment of the stomach. Although *H. pylori* is much more tolerant of an acid environment than most bacteria, it cannot proliferate in areas of high acid production so it is more likely to get a grip in people whose stomach acid secretions are declining, and those with gut inflammation, which further decreases stomach acid secretions (see Chapter 16).[2] Whether or not this bacterial infection is the original cause of digestive problems or the consequence of having an inflamed and aggravated digestive tract, there is little doubt that it makes matters much worse by reducing the body's production of protective gastric mucus, leading to inflammation and ulceration.[3] Being infected with helicobacter increases a person's risk of having a duodenal ulcer by five times,[4] and 95 per cent of people with duodenal ulcers are infected.

Therefore, anyone with ulceration, persistent indigestion or gastric pain is well advised to be tested for H. *pylori* infection. This involves a simple blood test, which your doctor can arrange for you. If the diagnosis is positive, conventional treatment involves specific antibiotics. There are, however, a wide range of natural alternatives and complementary medicines, which are discussed fully in Chapter 18.

Hiatus hernia

Another common cause of gastric pain and heartburn is having a hiatus hernia. Normally the stomach, which is located below the diaphragm muscle (see illustration on page 34), is closed off at either end by a circular muscle, thereby keeping the stomach acid contained; however, an estimated 50 per cent of people over the age of 50 have part of their stomach above the diaphragm muscle. This means that stomach acid can leak into the oesophagus, causing heartburn and gastric pain.

This physical defect, which can be relatively easily corrected, probably occurs for two reasons. The first is that the stomach can go into spasm when it is inflamed and irritated, and may end up dislocated. The other is a weakness in the diaphragm muscle (which is kept strong by deep breathing and exercise that stimulates deep breaths).

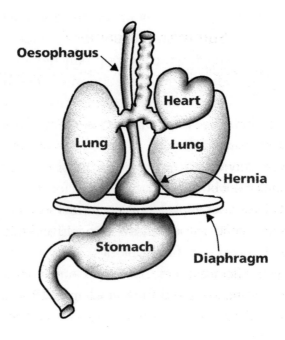

Hiatus hernia

Although it is said that having a genetically shorter oesophagus is a major cause, it is unlikely that this explains the
prevalence of the problem. It is possible that an oesophagus
in spasm could also pull the stomach up, again resulting in
a hiatus hernia. In any event there are physical techniques
practised by naturopaths and some osteopaths and kinesiologists that can help correct this condition. If muscle
spasm is involved, capsules of peppermint oil, which is a
muscle relaxant, can be beneficial (see Chapter 17 on irritable bowel syndrome).

Summary – Chapter 4

If you have acidity problems, indigestion, gastric pain or ulceration, follow these guidelines:

- If you have the symptoms of underacidity, supplement a digestive enzyme containing betaine hydrochloride (betaine HCl), plus 15mg of zinc. Or supplement betaine HCl on its own.
- Minimise your intake of gastric irritants such as aspirin, coffee, alcohol, very hot drinks and spicy food.
- If you suffer from overacidity, reduce your intake of concentrated protein-rich foods such as meat, fish and eggs, and have more vegetable proteins instead.
- If you have an ulcer, supplement omega-3 fats, 1g of calcium or magnesium ascorbate and 3,300mcg/10,000iu of vitamin A in the retinol form. You should also get yourself tested for *Helicobacter pylori*.

PART II

IMPROVING
ABSORPTION

CHAPTER 5

You Are What You Absorb

C ompletely digesting your food is one aspect of digestion – the other is being able to absorb it properly. So
far we've been talking about eating the correct foods
and digesting them down into the right-sized particles that
will be beneficial for the immune system. But does the food
you eat, once turned into nutrients, actually get through the
intestinal wall to nourish your body? The popular conception
is that, once your food is digested, it just passes through the
small intestine and into the body via the blood. In truth, however, there's much more to it than this. First of all, the small
intestine isn't small. Although only about 6m in length, it has
a surface area larger than a tennis court – about 200 times
the surface area of your skin. The highly active cells that line
this surface (the intestinal mucosa) are replaced on average
every four days. If this surface area isn't healthy, your ability
to absorb nutrients from food and your ability to reject toxic
substances won't be great either.

Different nutrients are absorbed through different sections of the small intestine, each requiring a different set
of conditions to maximise absorption. The duodenum,
for example, is just one step down from the stomach, so it

normally has a slightly acid environment, which helps the absorption of minerals, fats and B vitamins. A lack of stomach acid, perhaps due to zinc deficiency as suggested on page 29, can have the knock-on effect of reducing the amount of nutrients absorbed (ironically, zinc itself can be affected by this). As we have seen, vitamin B_{12} cannot be absorbed as such, but must first combine with intrinsic factor, which is produced in the stomach provided adequate stomach acid is secreted.

Other conditions also help absorption, such as the presence of the right kind of bacteria and fibre and the absence of digestive irritants, which are discussed in the following chapters. The two keys to maximising absorption, therefore, are keeping your digestive tract healthy and keeping the environment in there just right.

Promoting healthy absorption

The surface of the small intestine is made up of tiny protrusions called villi. These can be easily damaged by the consumption of fried food and alcohol, as well as by food allergies, irritating substances in food, and other factors, such as infections. When this happens, you get varying degrees of intestinal permeability, otherwise known as leaky gut syndrome.

The good news is that the intestinal mucosal cells, which line the villi, are among the most rapidly regenerating cells in the body. Supplying these cells with the right nutrients is a vital step towards maximising nutrient absorption. These nutrients include: vitamin A, which keeps the cell membrane strong and healthy; zinc, which is needed for repairing and replacing worn-out mucosal cells; glutamine, an amino acid, and butyric acid, a kind of fat, both of which act as fuel for the mucosal cells. All these nutrients help to promote healthy absorption.

Although almost all body cells run on glucose (the end product of digesting carbohydrate), the intestinal mucosa can feed off glutamine and butyric acid. Under normal conditions there is no need to eat butyric acid, as it is produced in the digestive tract by bacteria, particularly in the colon. Butyric acid levels are sometimes measured in stool tests to indicate the health of the colon. When levels are low, or when the digestive tract has become damaged and permeable, supplementing butyric acid can help restore digestive health (see Chapter 23). The same applies to the amino acid glutamine. Although not an essential nutrient as such, glutamine is certainly very helpful in nourishing, repairing and rebuilding the small intestine. It also strengthens immunity. Glutamine has also proven helpful for healing a damaged or permeable digestive tract, to aid recovery after surgery or after an infection.

If you have had a gastrointestinal infection, or have been taking antibiotics, or if you simply don't feel well nourished after a meal and suspect your absorption might not be up to scratch, you may benefit from supplementing 5–10g of glutamine. It is best, and generally much less expensive, to buy it as a powder. A heaped teaspoon is about 5g and should be taken with water, before going to bed. Use cold water, not hot, since heat destroys glutamine. This is akin to feeding your lawn: as you sleep, glutamine helps your mucosal cells to regenerate and repair. This is important because these mucosal cells not only control absorption but they also capture waste in the bloodstream, such as mucus, fat and toxins, and dump it into the digestive tract. It's a two-way street.

How absorption happens

Under a microscope your intestinal wall looks very much like a brick wall, each brick being a cell with tight junctions in between. Although some nutrients simply pass in between these cells into the body by diffusing across the intestinal wall, most are actively carried across by carrier molecules. The mechanism to open and close these junctions is carried out by a messenger molecule called zonulin. The level of zonulin, which opens up these junctions, is increased or decreased by the responses of the gut's highly active immune system, known as GALT (gut-associated lymphatic tissue) and also its nervous system. Both are checking out which nutrient can enter and which can't.

If a nutrient is beneficial and makes its way unhindered through this system, an appropriate absorption process, dependent on various nutrients, will carry the nutrient across. But a vicious circle can arise if absorption of nutrients is under par, because the consequent lack of nutrients will further impair absorption. Also, without proper digestion, incompletely digested food particles can trigger a reaction by the GALT.

Glucose and amino acids are the nutrients that need to be actively transported across the intestinal wall and are therefore the most susceptible to malabsorption. When the GALT reacts strongly against a food, such as wheat gluten in the case of a person with celiac disease, the net result is that the intestinal cells become damaged and the villi flatten out as they die off, until a person simply can't absorb sufficient nutrients and therefore wastes away.

An alternative scenario is one where the tight junctions get loose (creating what is known as 'leaky gut syndrome') and toxins and incompletely digested food molecules get

through, triggering the immune system to go ha'
resulting 'red alert' state is known as inflamm\a
can become systemic, resulting in aching joints,
problems, itchy skin, headaches and/or chroni\
Wheat, which contains a type of gluten called gliadin,
promotes a leaky gut by triggering a release of zonulin.[1]
Bacterial imbalances can too. I'll explain how to reverse
gut inflammation in Chapter 16 and how to heal a leaky
gut in Chapter 15.

The above types of scenario underlie so many of the digestive and non-digestive complaints that people frequently
suffer from in the 21st century.

Setting up the right conditions

Before food can be absorbed it must first be prepared
for absorption. As well as involving digestive enzymes,
this process also requires enzymes that promote active
absorption.

These are dependent on nutrients – in other words, certain
nutrients help other nutrients to be absorbed. An example is
zinc and vitamin B_6: this was demonstrated in an experiment
in which animals were given increasing amounts of vitamin
B_6 and the same amount of zinc. The more B_6 they were given,
the more zinc they absorbed into the bloodstream.[2]

Some minerals, such as zinc and selenium, compete with
each other for absorption, so technically they are better
absorbed individually, on an empty stomach. However,
unless you fancy swallowing supplements at several different times throughout the day, for practical purposes it
is fine to do what nature does – take in nutrients as part of
food. But bear in mind that certain foods contain substances

that can interfere with the absorption of nutrients. These include:

- Phytates in wheat, whole grains, nuts, seeds and beans[3]
- Oxalates in spinach and rhubarb
- Methylxanthines in tea, coffee and cocoa

The effect of these substances on the absorption of nutrients is not minor; for example, when you eat kale you absorb approximately 40 per cent of the iron within it; however, when you eat spinach, especially rich in oxalates, you absorb something in the region of 5 per cent. Cooking spinach helps a bit but don't rely on spinach for iron. Drinking a cup of coffee with a meal can also reduce iron absorption to a third. My recommendation is to only drink coffee on its own, not with food, if at all.

Phytates can be both good and bad. A phytate is phytic acid (a source of phosphorus) bound to a mineral. Phytates are in the highest amounts in whole foods and the lowest in refined foods. They tend to break down with cooking, soaking and during the fermenting of foods. On the one hand they make minerals less available but, on the other, they are found in whole foods, which are naturally higher in minerals and, in reality, most will be broken down during food preparation. Vitamin C also helps to enhance mineral absorption, counteracting the effect of phytates. If, for example, you soak nuts overnight, you reduce their phytate content but this doesn't affect their mineral levels.

Any substance that irritates the digestive tract – from alcohol to antibiotics – will also have undesirable effects on absorption. There's a chart at www.patrickholford.com/maximisingabsorption that shows you what helps and what hinders the absorption of nutrients.

Testing your absorption

If your healthcare practitioner suspects that you might not be absorbing properly, he or she is likely to run a stool analysis, which can measure the presence of proteins, fats and carbohydrates in the stool, indicating a compromised ability to digest or absorb your food.

A more specific indicator of absorption problems is an intestinal permeability test. This involves drinking something and then collecting a urine sample. This is then analysed to indicate what sizes of molecule are passing through the wall of your digestive tract.

Therapeutic strategies for correcting identified absorption problems are outlined in Chapter 15.

Summary – Chapter 5

Unless you have an identified absorption problem, the following guidelines can help you to maximise your ability to absorb nutrients from your food:

- If you drink tea, coffee or alcohol, don't take it with meals.
- Don't eat too much modern wheat (see Chapter 9 for more on this).
- Supplement a high-strength multivitamin and mineral, providing at least 7,500iu (2,275mg) of vitamin A and 15mg of zinc, and take your supplements with food. Supplement one teaspoon (5g) of glutamine dissolved in cold water before bed for a week to improve gut wall integrity.

CHAPTER 6

The Fibre Factor

We all owe a lot of our knowledge about the importance of fibre to Drs Denis Burkitt and Hubert Trowell, who painstakingly travelled the world collecting stool samples. The conclusion of their research was that communities with loose-formed stools had very low incidences of colitis, diverticulitis, appendicitis, haemorrhoids and constipation, whereas communities with hardened, compacted stools were plagued by such digestive diseases, as well as the classic Western diseases of diabetes, heart disease and cancer. Burkitt and Trowell identified the health-promoting food ingredient as fibre.

What is fibre?

Not all types of carbohydrate can be digested and broken down into glucose as fuel for the body. Indigestible carbohydrate is called fibre. In recent years some kinds of starches, not previously classified as fibre, have been found to be resistant to digestion. They are called 'resistant starches', and by and large they act in the same way as fibre (more of this on page 57).

Fibre is a natural constituent of a healthy diet that is high in fruit, vegetables, lentils, beans and whole grains. If you eat such a diet you have less risk of bowel cancer, diabetes or diverticular disease, and you are unlikely to suffer from constipation.

Contrary to the popular image of fibre as mere roughage, it can absorb water. As it does so, it makes faecal matter bulkier, less dense and easier to pass along the digestive tract. This decreases the amount of time food waste spends inside the body and reduces the risk of infection or cell changes due to carcinogens that are produced when some foods, particularly meat, degrade. Bulkier faecal matter also means less chance of a blockage, or constipation.

There are many different kinds of fibre, some of which are proteins, not carbohydrates. Some fibre, such as that found in oats, is called 'soluble fibre' and combines with sugar molecules to slow down the absorption of carbohydrates. This type, therefore, helps to keep blood sugar levels balanced, which means that you have a more even energy and control over your weight.

Some types of fibre are much more water-absorbent than others. Whereas wheat fibre, for example, swells to ten times its original volume in water, glucomannan fibre (from the Japanese konjac plant) swells to 100 times its volume in water. Highly absorbent types of fibre, by bulking up foods and slowing down the release of sugars, can help to control the appetite and they also play a part in weight maintenance.

How much fibre do we need?

The average daily intake of fibre in people in the UK and the US is about 20g, which is less than half that of rural Africans, who consume around 55g a day and suffer from few of the lower digestive tract diseases so common in the West. An ideal intake of fibre is not less than 35g a day. The chart below shows you how much of each food you would need to eat to get 10g of fibre; for example, if you have a cup of oats (240ml by volume), an apple and a heaped tablespoonful of seeds for breakfast, this will provide 10g + 3g + 2g = 15g of fibre. A large salad containing crunchy vegetables, such as carrots, cabbage or broccoli pieces, might give you a further 15g. A meal based on beans, lentils or peas is likely to provide a further 15g.

Amount of food required to supply 10g of fibre

Food	Amount (for equivalent of 10g grain fibre)
Almonds	107g/⅛ cup*
Apple	500g/3–4 apples
Apricots, dried	42g/1 cup*
Baked beans	137g/1 small can
Baked potato (skin on)	400g/1 large
Bananas	625g/3 bananas
Broccoli	358g/1 large head
Cabbage	466g/1 medium
Carrots	310g/3 carrots
Cauliflower	475g/1 large
Coleslaw	400g/1 large serving
Cornflakes	91g/3½ cups*
Figs, dried	54g/⅓ cup*

Food	Amount (for equivalent of 10g grain fibre)
Lentils, cooked	270g/2 cups*
New potatoes, boiled	500g/7 potatoes
Oatcakes	250g/10 biscuits
Oats	75g/1 cup*
Oranges	415g/3 oranges
Peaches	625g/6 peaches
Peanuts	125g/1 cup*
Peas	83g/1 cup*
Prunes	146g/1 cup
Rice crispies	222g/8 cups
Rye bread	160g/6 slices
Sunflower seeds	147g/1 cup*
Wheat bran	23g/½ cup*
White bread	370g/15 slices
Wholemeal bread	115g/5 slices

*1 cup = 240ml by volume

Provided the right foods are eaten, 35g of fibre can easily be achieved without the need to add extra. Professor of Nutrition John Dickerson, from the University of Surrey, has stressed the danger of simply adding wheat bran to a nutrient-poor diet. The reason for this is that wheat bran contains high levels of phytate, which reduces the absorption of essential minerals, including zinc. Overall, it is probably best to get a mixture of fibre from oats, lentils, beans, seeds, fruits and raw or lightly cooked vegetables. Much of the fibre in vegetables is destroyed by cooking, so vegetables are best eaten crunchy.

Fibre, soluble fibre and the constipation myth

Popular advice for constipation is to drink more water and eat more fibre-rich foods such as whole grains. These are more fad than fact, however, since there is no consistent evidence that fibre works, nor water. In fact, in some studies having more fibre makes matters worse, not better. Once you are constipated, adding a lot of fibre in the form of whole grains and then drinking a lot of water is not proven to be effective, although drinking sufficient water *on a daily basis* helps you to avoid constipation.

In a study of 63 adults who suffered from chronic constipation and who had been on a high-fibre diet and/or were taking fibre supplements, 41 were put on a no-fibre diet, 16 on a reduced-fibre diet and 4 remained on their high-fibre diet.[4] Of those put on the no-fibre diet, frequency went from once every 3.75 days to once a day. Those on the reduced-fibre diet went from once every 4.19 days to every 1.9 days, and there was no change in those who stayed on their high-fibre diet.

This study is one of several that show no benefit, or worsening, on a high-fibre diet. A review of studies treating IBS sufferers with high-fibre diets shows much the same thing, with an increase in regular 'insoluble' fibres found in wholegrain wheat probably making matters worse, not better.[5] Evidence of their benefit in studies of people with IBS is rather thin.[6]

Most studies do, however, show a benefit for 'soluble' fibres.[7] These are found in oats and chia seeds. Flax seeds or linseeds, in contrast, contain insoluble fibre. People given soluble fibres in studies were almost twice as likely to report a benefit, with increased frequency and ease, than those on a placebo.

One way to get soluble fibres is to have a tablespoon of chia seeds a day, which is what I do. Another is to eat whole oat products. You can further increase your soluble fibre intake by adding a teaspoon of oat bran to cereal.

Soluble fibres are also found in vegetables, although they are somewhat destroyed by heat and prolonged cooking. They behave quite differently to, for example, wheat fibre.

Soluble fibres reduce hunger and help you to lose weight

Soluble fibres dissolve and become gel-like, absorbing lots of water, unlike wheat bran, for example, which absorbs very little. The best-known example of a soluble fibre is oat fibre or bran, which is rich in a type of fibre called beta-glucans. When beta-glucans is added to or cooked with water it becomes viscous; this is what gives porridge its smooth consistency. This soluble fibre helps to coat foods and the digestive tract in a way that slows down the release of sugars from food. It also attaches to cholesterol in the gut and helps to eliminate it. Generally speaking, the more water-absorbing and viscous a food, the better. This also makes you feel fuller so you naturally eat less.

Barley is another example of a food that is exceptionally high in soluble fibres that help to stabilise your blood sugar level. Other common soluble fibres in foods include pectin, which is particularly high in citrus fruit and apples, and algin in seaweed.

There are also some food sources that you are unlikely to have come across, such as konjac fibre, which is a potato-like tuber found in Japan, psyllium husks, guar gum and xanthan gum. In Japan you can find dishes made with konjac fibre but they're not on the menu in the West. These ingredients are often used as thickeners in foods and can also be used to create 'super-fibres' that you can buy as powders or capsules or in special shake mixes. These are all designed to help stabilise your blood sugar levels, which, as we have seen, is important because it is the effect of blood sugar spikes that causes excess sugar to be dumped into the liver and then to be turned into fat, making you gain weight, especially around the middle. These products are well worth knowing about because taking a capsule before a meal, or a spoonful dissolved in water, makes a massive difference to the glycemic load (the speed at which carbohydrate is released) of the meal you are about to eat. (See the box opposite.)

Glucomannan and PGX – super fibres

One of my favourite fibres, widely used in Asia but not in the UK, is glucomannan, the soluble fibre in konjac. Glucomannan absorbs 50 times more water than wheat bran, bulking up the food you eat and making you feel fuller for longer. Because of its highly absorbent properties, it is very important to take it with a lot of water. This highly absorbent property means two things: it helps to eliminate cholesterol by binding to it in the digestive tract, but the real gold of glucomannan is its ability to help to balance your blood sugar. A study in Thailand found that taking 1g of glucomannan before meals significantly lowered the glycemic load, or the effect on the body's insulin levels (see the box opposite), and the need for insulin, in people with type-2 diabetes.[8] Other studies have shown that glucomannan lowers cholesterol[9] and also stabilises blood sugar,[10] which is associated with improving insulin sensitivity.

The glycemic load and the benefit of low-GL foods

The glycemic load is a unit of measurement that tells you exactly what a particular food will do to your blood sugar. It is often written as GL. Foods with a high GL have a greater effect on your blood sugar, which isn't desirable. Foods with a low GL, on the other hand, encourage the body to burn fat.

When your blood sugar level increases, the hormone insulin is released into the bloodstream to remove the glucose (sugar). Some glucose goes to the brain and muscles where it's used as an energy fuel, but any excess goes to the liver where it's turned into fat and stored, causing you to gain weight. Insulin is known as the fat-storing hormone.

The glycemic load is based on the glycemic index (GI). Put simply, the glycemic index of a food tells you whether the carbohydrate in a food is fast or slow releasing (fast is bad, slow is good). What it doesn't tell you is exactly how much of the food is carbohydrate. The glycemic load, on the other hand, tells you both the type and the amount of carbohydrate in a food and what that particular carbohydrate does to your blood sugar.

A low-GL diet Keeping your blood sugar balanced is the concept at the heart of a low-GL diet – allowing sustainable weight loss. But it's also important in relation to digestion, because those low-GL foods are also beneficial to the gut. They include a wide range of non-starchy vegetables such as peppers, leafy greens, cauliflower, tomatoes, courgettes, mushrooms and aubergines. Low-GL foods also include those starchy vegetables that are slow-releasing. Here are some examples of low- and high-GL foods. Each item represents 10GLs, but you will see that you get a far greater quantity from the low-GL foods than you do from those in the list of high-GL foods:

Low-GL	High-GL
2 large punnets of strawberries	2 dates
6 oatcakes	1 slice of white bread
4 bowls of oat flakes	1 bowl of cornflakes
A large bowl of peanuts	A packet of crisps
1 pint of tomato juice	Half a glass of Lucozade
6 tablespoons of xylitol	2 teaspoons of honey
10 handfuls of green beans	10 French fries

In order to control blood sugar (and to lose weight, if that is also what you need), you need to limit your main meals to 10GLs and your snacks to 5GLs. If you do not need to lose weight you will be able to have 15GLs for your main meals. The recipes later in this book are based on this low-GL principle. (You can see a full list of foods in my books *The Low-GL Diet Bible* or *The Low-GL Diet Counter.*)

When you follow a low-GL diet you will be getting plenty of soluble fibre, which both improves gut transit time so that you don't become blocked up, and helps nourish healthy gut bacteria. Also, the low sugar levels in a low-GL diet prevent the growth of harmful bacteria and pathogens.

Glucomannan is also a brilliant aid for healthy weight loss. Two studies, one in Japan[11] and one in the US,[12] reported an additional 500g weight loss a week when patients took 3g of glucomannan a day. At the Institute for Optimum Nutrition, which I founded in 1984 to research what optimum nutrition really means and to train nutritional therapists, we decided to put glucomannan to the test by giving 3g a day to ten overweight people over a three-month period.[13] None made any apparent change to their diet or exercise regime. Nine completed the trial, with an average weight loss of 3kg each. A review of all studies to date in 2015, confirms that glucomannan is effective for weight loss in otherwise healthy, obese or overweight adults.[14] You need about 3g, or a flat teaspoon, for this kind of effect. These days it is hard for food manufacturers to make any health claims for their foods unless they have been through the extremely rigorous process of proving the claim with the European Food Safety Authority (EFSA). Glucomannan is one of few natural remedies that have been allowed a weight-loss claim. The EFSA concluded that 'a cause and effect relationship has been established between the consumption of glucomannan and the reduction of body weight in the context of an energy-restricted diet', provided that at least 3g of glucomannan is consumed daily. It also contributes to maintaining normal cholesterol levels at a dose of 4g daily.

Every morning, just before my breakfast, I take three Carboslow capsules (which contain glucomannan) with a large glass of water, especially on days when I'm not eating a high soluble fibre breakfast (such as scrambled eggs and salmon rather than oats, chia seeds and berries). The net result is no hunger until lunchtime. I find it a useful curb on my otherwise voracious appetite. If I wanted to lose weight, I'd do the same just before lunch and dinner. This adds about 1 litre of water, absorbed by the soluble fibres, into the contents moving through the digestive tract, which can be really helpful if you don't go to the toilet regularly and suffer with constipation. I would caution, however, to always have glucomannan with a large glass of water and to start gradually, just taking it once a day before breakfast, for example, and building up to two or three times a day over a couple of weeks. This has proven helpful in one study with adults prone to constipation, both increasing frequency and ease.[15]

PGX

Exceptional results have also been demonstrated for a special type of fibre rich in glucomannan called PGX, which is a big seller in the US but not yet available in the UK. It is the most highly water-absorbing fibre, created by reacting glucomannan with other plant fibres (alginate from seaweed, and xanthan gum) to make it more viscous. PGX is a powder and is also available in capsules. Taking a heaped teaspoon (5g) in a glass of water two or three times a day before meals reduces appetite and substantially reduces the glycemic load of the meal you are about to eat.[16]

In a study by Professor Jenny Brand-Miller from the University of Sydney, who has been very instrumental in promoting the value of low-GL eating, she found that taking 5g of PGX powder with water before, with or immediately after breakfast cut the GL of the meal by around a quarter.[17] This means that adding the PGX effectively lowers the GI or GL of the glucose,[18] which illustrates the importance of having a soluble-fibre-rich diet for blood sugar control. The GL-lowering effect is even greater when added to a meal; for example, if you take a teaspoonful of PGX with a meal containing a serving of rice you will dramatically stabilise the blood sugar spike of the meal, turning it from a mountain into a rolling hill.[19] This is almost equivalent to halving the GL of the meal. In another study, taking PGX almost halved the feelings of hunger before a meal and the appetite, measured by the quantity of food desired.[20]

Resistant starch

Some kinds of starch or carbohydrate are difficult to digest and act as fibre. These 'resistant' starches also feed gut bacteria and are thus called prebiotics because they can help healthy bacteria in the gut to grow.[21] A classic prebiotic is FOS (fructo-oligosaccharides), which you might have seen in the list of ingredients of probiotic supplements. They are included to feed the bacteria when they hit fluids in your digestive tract. Another is inulin (containing fructans), derived from chicory root. Oats contains glucans, a similar molecule.

Having a diet high in resistant starch is a good idea, and there are two ways to do this. The first is to eat foods that are naturally high in it. These include:

Jerusalem artichokes
Garlic, leeks and onions – in that order
Asparagus
Cashew nuts
Oats, uncooked
Chicory
Green bananas, raw
Peas, beans and lentils

The second way to increase your intake of resistant starch is to cook a carb and cool it, then to eat it cold or reheated. Oats naturally have ten times more resistant starch raw than cooked, but if you make porridge and cool it, you recreate resistant starch. I sometimes do this, leaving my excess porridge in the fridge to eat as a snack.

The same is true with potatoes, rice and pasta. If you steam new potatoes, then cool them, to make a potato salad, you massively increase the level of resistant starch. You can do the same thing with rice and pasta, but it is best to start with a long-grain brown rice or whole Kamut pasta (see page 92), which is naturally high in resistant starch; for example, you could make a pasta salad or a cold rice pudding using dried Montmorency cherries instead of raisins, and oat milk instead of cow's milk, if you are dairy sensitive.

Even though the sugar in bananas is fast-releasing, hence they are high GL, the same is not true for a green banana eaten raw. Sometimes I cut a green banana into thirds then put half of one-third, plus some frozen blueberries, in my breakfast smoothie mix in the morning.

Chicory root – a source of inulin

Chicory root is especially high in a resistant starch called inulin. Quoting the European Food Safety Authority (EFSA), 'Six out of eight human studies provided reported an increase in stool frequency with the consumption of "native chicory inulins" or chicory inulin.' No adverse effects have been reported in any of these studies. This claim can be made if the food given provides 12g of inulin, roughly two teaspoons. It is naturally sweet but doesn't raise your blood sugar levels at all because it isn't absorbed. Only the bacteria in your gut can digest it.

The other big advantage of resistant starches is that by feeding healthy bacteria in the gut they help these bacteria to produce short-chain fatty acids, especially butyrate, which is extremely good for colon health, helping to reduce the risk of cancer, speeding up the metabolism and reducing inflammation.

Inulin, which is derived from chicory root powder, has another advantage. Its natural sweetness means it can be used as a sweetener, but it has zero GLs (the measure used for the speed at which carbohydrates are released in the body, thereby affecting blood sugar levels). It is one of my favourite natural sweeteners, another being xylitol, which is derived from xylose, the predominant sugar in berries, cherries and plums.

Are there any downsides?

If you consume too much resistant starch, there are two side effects, which are more apparent in some people than others. The first is flatulence. When bacteria in the gut feed off resistant starch they can produce gas. This is very much a quantity effect, and different people have different sensitivities to these foods. I know many sensitive people who have no problem as long as they simultaneously supplement digestive enzymes.

The other remote possibility is that, if you have a gut infection caused by unfriendly gut bacteria, a high intake of prebiotics will feed the bad bacteria too. It is better, therefore, to have some probiotics; however, if you feed good bacteria, they tend to crowd out bad bacteria, so the net effect is usually positive in any case.

The other potential problem is increased 'frequency'. Of course, for many this is a benefit. The same is true with foods high in xylose, such as plums or prunes. In a way, this is a good natural indicator that your body has consumed more than your system is perhaps designed for; however, for some people with IBS, increasing resistant starch makes them feel worse. A low-FODMAP diet (see Chapter 23), which helps some people with IBS, specifically avoids foods with resistant starch. We are all different and have different sensitivities, so one man's food will be another man's poison, but if you are not one of those people who has difficulty with resistant starches, they can have many healthy benefits for you.

Testing gastrointestinal transit time

One of the great advantages of having a diet high in soluble fibres and resistant starches is that it increases your gastrointestinal transit time (the time it takes for food to pass through your digestive tract), reducing the amount of time food has to putrefy in the intestines. Apart from analysing what you eat, you can get a 'functional' indication of whether or not you're getting enough fibre by doing a very simple test to measure your gastrointestinal transit time. Either buy some charcoal tablets and take 20 grains (or 1g), or eat a whole beetroot. Note the time and date you do this. When you see a darkened stool, in the case of the charcoal, or a reddened stool, in the case of the beetroot, you can calculate your transit time.

If your transit time is less than 12 hours, you might not be absorbing all the nutrients from your food, and you should investigate the possibility of absorption problems (see Chapter 5). If your transit time is more than 24 hours, this indicates that waste material is spending too long inside you, a factor that increases your risk of colon-related diseases. This is a signal to increase your fibre intake and take some exercise, which strengthens the abdominal muscles.

Exercise helps because it promotes deeper breathing so that the diaphragm (a dome-shaped muscle that separates the chest and abdominal cavity) is pulled down to allow for a deeper inhalation, and released as you exhale. This action massages the digestive tract and promotes bowel movements.

Drinking sufficient water is also part of the equation. If you don't drink enough water, the contents of your digestive tract are likely to become less watery and consequently harder to move along. However, drinking tons of water has not been shown to be effective in treating constipation. Increasing soluble fibre, and drinking *enough* water, works better. The oils and fibres in ground seeds, such as flax and chia seeds, also help to promote healthy bowel motions. I prefer chia seeds because of their higher soluble-fibre content.

Summary – Chapter 6

To keep everything moving along:

- Eat wholefoods – whole grains, lentils, beans, nuts, seeds, fresh fruit and vegetables.
- Avoid refined, white, processed and overcooked foods.
- Eat vegetables every day, raw or lightly cooked.
- Eat foods rich in resistant starch – garlic, leeks and onions, asparagus, cashew nuts, raw oats, peas, beans and lentils.
- Use xylitol or chicory root powder (inulin) as a sweetener.
- Take a tablespoonful of chia seeds.
- Eat whole oats, as oat flakes or rough oatcakes.
- Take a teaspoon or three capsules of Carboslow or PGX, or glucomannan, with a large glass of water, with meals up to three times a day.
- Exercise at least three times a week.
- Drink plenty of water – at least 1.5 litres a day.

CHAPTER 7

How to Promote
Healthy Intestinal Flora

D id you know that up to 2kg of your body weight is bacteria? The average person has about 130 different types of friendly bacteria, mainly resident in the digestive tract, which are forever multiplying.[22] There are about 100 trillion bacteria in your digestive tract, most of which are in the colon.[23] That's more than the total number of cells in your body. Every day you make quantities of bacteria and eliminate an equal amount in stools.

Not all of these bacteria are good for you, but, provided you have enough of the health-promoting bacteria, they act as your first line of defence against unfriendly bacteria and other disease-producing microbes, including viruses and fungi.

The good bacteria make some vitamins and digest fibre, allowing you to derive more nutrients from otherwise indigestible food, and also help to promote a healthy digestive environment.

It is not just the quality but also the quantity of bacteria that make a difference to your health – and the balance between bacteria in the small intestine and the large intestine. Too many of the wrong kind of bacteria in the small intestine leads to too much fermentation and gas production. This is called small intestine bacterial overgrowth (SIBO) and is often present in people who have irritable bowel syndrome (IBS). This can be detected by a breath test that measures how much of the exhalation is methane or hydrogen. A nutritional therapist might recommend this test if they suspect SIBO. For these people, lots of prebiotics and resistant starches, as discussed in the last chapter, will not be a good idea.

We are, in fact, partly descended from bacteria. Within our body cells are organelles (or components), each with a specific function. Biologists now believe that the complex cells that make up our bodies may have developed from smaller micro-organisms, such as bacteria, working together. Over time, this cooperation led to the development of the complex cells from which we are made; for example, the energy factories within our cells (called mitochondria) are derived from bacteria.

A healthy or diseased microbiome

Like our fingerprints, our microbiome (the specific family of microorganisms found in our gut) is unique to each one of us and is comprised of a balance of different bacteria, some better for us than others. What exactly makes up a healthy microbiome is the subject of much research. This research tends to focus either on specific strains of bacteria and their effects on specific diseases or, more recently, the difference between the microbiome in healthy people and that in sick people. (This is confusingly often called the microbiota – microbiome referring to the gene pool of all the bacteria, rather than the actual tribe of bacteria.)

Several studies have reported a different balance of gut bacteria, or microbiota, associated with diabetes, inflammatory bowel disorders, asthma, mental illness and obesity, with more pathogenic bacteria and fewer healthy ones. But is this difference a *cause* of the disease or a *consequence*, perhaps of a bad diet that then leads to the disease?

Slim people, for example, have a different microbiota to obese people, which begs the question as to whether the microbiota of slim people could be keeping them slim. Such a cause and effect has not yet been established, but the first human trial, giving 21 obese people poo pills from slim people is underway at Massachusetts General Hospital in the US. This follows a study in 2013 that suggested a possible cause-and-effect relationship between gut microbes and the prevention of obesity. Four sets of human twins, where one twin was a healthy weight and the other was obese, donated their microbe profile to mice. The mice who received an obese twin's microbes gained weight, regardless of their diet.

The 'poo' shock value is nothing new. When probiotics were first touted back in the 1980s, I remember a newspaper headline that read 'Let them eat shit', ridiculing the use of human strains of gut bacteria for the treatment of disease. The big question the poo pill study hopes to answer is whether slimmer people's bacterial signature is simply a consequence of a better diet, and one that keeps them slim, or whether the bacteria in themselves have any impact on weight gain, appetite or metabolism. A likely benefit, if there is any, might be attributable to larger quantities of probiotics, or beneficial bacteria, in slimmer, healthier people.

As gross as this might sound, the impact our microbiota – that is the unique signature of gut bacteria – has on health and metabolism is certainly a worthy subject of growing interest in medical research.

Supplementing probiotics

A more acceptable approach for many is to supplement specific strains of beneficial bacteria, also known as probiotics. The principal friendly bacteria include the families of *Lactobacillus* and *Bifidus* bacteria. The *Bifidus* family of bacteria generally makes up a quarter of the total flora in the digestive tract.

The first controlled study on a particular strain of *Lactobacillus* bacteria reported a significant reduction in BMI and a 4.6 per cent reduction in abdominal fat after 12 weeks.[24] Another study in 2014, published in the *British Journal of Nutrition*[25], and using *Lactobacillus rhamnosus*, reported a small weight loss in women and none in men, compared to placebo, after 12 weeks.

The most recent study in the *American Journal of Clinical Nutrition* compared the effect of giving a probiotic yoghurt or a standard low-fat yoghurt to 89 overweight women. The women were randomly assigned to either consume probiotic yoghurt daily or regular yoghurt, for 12 weeks. All were following the same calorie-controlled diet. There were no significant weight-loss differences between the two groups.[26] To date I would not say there is anything compelling to recommend the use of probiotics for weight loss.

Research into other disease states, based on changes in the microbiota, is just beginning. A study last year, giving a combination of *Lactobacillus acidophilus* and *Bifidobacterium bifidum* to 60 pregnant women with gestational diabetes, reported a decrease in glucose and insulin levels compared to placebo.[27] This confirms other findings that gut bacteria alter how we process sugars in our diet.

Taking supplements of these friendly bacteria also gives pathogenic (harmful) bacteria less chance of survival and has proven effective in reducing symptoms of infectious diseases that induce symptoms such as diarrhoea.

There are many different strains of friendly bacteria, some of which actually live in the gut, whereas others simply pass through but are useful while they're there. Here are some of the different types:

The principal friendly bacteria

	Children	Adults
Resident	B. infantis	L. acidophilus
	B. bifidum	L. rhamnosus
	B. bacterium	B. longum
		L. salivarius enterococci
Passing through	L. bulgaricus	L. casei (from cheese)
	S. thermophilus	S. thermophilus
		S. salivarius
		L. salivarius
		L. bulgaricus

Key: B. = Bifidobacterium; L. = Lactobacillus; S. = Streptococcus

Those bacteria that are resident, sometimes called 'human strain', are usually better at fighting infection because they multiply and colonise the digestive tract. Others are available in fermented foods, such as yoghurt, miso and sauerkraut. Yoghurt and other fermented dairy products often contain *Streptococcus thermophilus* or *L. bulgaricus*. These bacteria will be present for a week or so, doing good work. They, like the other beneficial bacteria, can make vitamins as well as turning lactose (the main sugar in milk) into lactic acid. This makes the digestive tract slightly more acidic, which inhibits disease-causing microbes such as *Candida albicans* from multiplying. Drinks made with bacteria or yeasts, such as kefir (see page 72) and kombucha are becoming increasingly popular among the health conscious. Another yeast, *Saccharomyces boulardii*, is proving helpful for those with candidiasis (see Chapter 22) and in combating other infections, as well as stimulating growth of the beneficial immunoglobulin, secretory IgA, which helps to fight off invaders. (More about secretory IgA on page 122.)

There are many other strains touted for various health benefits. For some strains of bacteria, used in probiotic drinks, the drink makers have managed to obtain a patent. I prefer, when recommending probiotics, to stick to the human strains of bacteria, which cannot be patented because they already exist in the natural environment of our gut.

Bacteria benefits

The benefits of having a healthy population of beneficial bacteria are many and include:

- Making vitamins, including vitamins B_1, B_2, B_3, B_5, B_6, B_{12}, biotin, vitamins A and K as well as short-chain fatty acids. One study found 50 per cent higher levels of B_{12} in those people who were supplementing probiotics after gastric bypass surgery.[28]
- Ensuring normal function of the intestine, including motility, secretion of mucus and absorption as well as helping to eliminate cholesterol and bile.[29]

- Helping to digest carbohydrates and proteins, such as casein and gluten, and digesting lactose and other carbohydrates.[30]
- Fighting infections: they have been shown to halve recovery time from diarrhoea and prevent the overgrowth of salmonella, *E. coli* (responsible for many cases of food poisoning), *Helicobacter pylori* and *Candida albicans*. Several studies have shown that some of the *Lactobacillus* strains can improve the effectiveness of flu vaccinations.[31]
- Boosting your immunity by increasing the number of immune cells and the production of secretory IgA.
- Promoting other 'good' bacteria, while reducing 'bad' bacteria. *Lactobacillus acidophilus* supplementation, for example, has been shown to promote the beneficial bifidobacteria and inhibit disease-producing microbes.[32]
- Repairing and promoting the health of the digestive tract and gut-wall integrity by enhancing 'tight-junction' stability (as explained on page 42).[33] Probiotics also ferment sugars into short-chain fatty acids,[34] such as butyric acid, which is used as fuel by the intestinal lining, helping it to repair itself.
- Reducing inflammation and allergic inflammatory reactions by inhibiting pro-inflammatory cytokine production, which is one of the key substances produced in the body that triggers pain.[35] A healthy population thus helps conditions such as arthritis[36] by lessening the response in the gut to allergenic foods.[37] Many food reactions might not be solely due to food allergy but also due to the feeding of unfriendly bacteria, which then produce substances that activate the immune system in the gut.[38]

Which conditions benefit the most from probiotics?

To date the conditions that have been helped by probiotic supplements and the specific strains of bacteria that have been used are as follows:

Condition	Most effective
Antibiotic-associated diarrhoea (AAD)	*Lactobacillus rhamnosus* or *Saccharomyces boulardii*
Clostridium difficile disease (CDD)	Combo of *Lactobacillus* and *Bifidobacterium*
Helicobacter pylori positive (HPP)	Combo of *Lactobacillus* and *Bifidobacterium*
Irritable bowel syndrome (IBS)	Combo of *Lactobacillus* and *Bifidobacterium*
Infectious diarrhoea (ID)	Combo of *Lactobacillus* and *Bifidobacterium*
Traveller's diarrhoea	*Lactobacillus acidophilus*
Pouchitis	Combo of *Lactobacillus* and *Bifidobacterium*
Inflammatory bowel disease	Combo of *Lactobacillus* and *Bifidobacterium* and *L. salivarius*
Eczema	Combo of *Lactobacillus* and *Bifidobacterium*
Allergic tendency	Combo of *Lactobacillus* and *Bifidobacterium*
Weight loss	Combo of *Lactobacillus* and *Bifidobacterium*

Condition	Most effective
Diabetes	Combo of *Lactobacillus* and *Bifidobacterium*
Candidiasis	Combo of *Lactobacillus* and *Bifidobacterium* and *Saccharomyces boulardii*

Different strains have been used for treating and testing the effects against different kinds of infections and digestive disorders. These include:

- *Lactobacillus* bacteria such as *L. rhamnosus* GG (LGG), *L. acidophilus, L. casei, L. plantarium, L. salivarius*
- Bifidobacteria such as *B. lactis* and *B. infantis*
- *Saccharomyces boulardii*
- *Clostridium butyricum*
- *Enterococcus faecium*
- *Streptococcus salivarius*

The most evidence exists for combinations of *Lactobacillus* and *Bifidobacterium*. Some of the special strains of bacteria are the most beneficial for children. These include *Bifidobacterium infantis*. Good for both adults and children is *Lactobacillus salivarius*, which attaches to the intestinal wall and has been shown to reduce the number of pathogenic organisms.[39]

A review of 23 studies on antibiotic-associated diarrhoea concluded that 'Moderate quality evidence suggests a protective effect of probiotics in preventing diarrhoea.' In this study, taking probiotics halved the incidence, and one person out of ten experienced a significant improvement. Among the various probiotics evaluated, *Lactobacillus rhamnosus* and *Saccharomyces boulardii* at 5–40 billion colony-forming units per day were particularly effective, with extremely rare adverse effects.[40]

How you can promote healthy bacteria

Many cultures have observed the health-promoting effects of fermented foods and include them as a regular part of their diet. These foods include:

- Yoghurt, cottage cheese, kefir (from dairy produce)
- Sauerkraut, pickles (from vegetables)
- Miso, tofu, natto, tempeh, tamari, shoyu, soya yoghurt (from soya)
- Sourdough bread (from Kamut or rye, assuming you are not sensitive to wheat or gluten)

Including these foods in your diet is a good way to promote healthy intestinal flora. So too is eating foods rich in resistant starch that feed the intestinal flora. The best food for health-promoting bacteria is something called fructo-oligosaccharides (or FOS for short), which I discussed on page 57 and are sometimes known as a prebiotic. Green bananas are especially rich in these, as are oats, garlic, Jerusalem artichokes and onions. One study found that eating banana powder thickened the stomach lining.[41]

Overall, eating a plant-based diet that is high in fruits and vegetables (which are naturally high in resistant starch) is much more likely to encourage healthy bacteria. On the other hand, a high-meat diet, apart from being the primary source of gastrointestinal infections, is more likely to introduce toxic breakdown products as well as slowing down gastrointestinal transit time. Eaten occasionally, with plenty of fibrous foods, meat is not a problem, but meat-based diets, with few fibrous foods and vegetables, increases the risk of digestive problems, including colorectal cancer. I'd aim for fish three times a week and meat a maximum of twice. If you do function well on a higher meat diet, make sure that it is organic lean meat, eaten with plenty of fibre-rich vegetables.

Kefir – make your own probiotics

My favourite food, or drink, for promoting a healthy microbiota is kefir. It has been drunk for hundreds of years as an elixir of life in the Caucasus mountains bordering Russia, Georgia and Azerbaijan and is made by adding kefir 'grains' – a symbiotic culture of bacteria and yeasts – into either milk or water with added sugar, to feed the kefir. It converts the sugar, or the lactose in the milk, into lactic acid and tastes quite tart and a little fizzy. This fermented drink contains a wide variety of yeasts and bacteria including numerous strains of *Lactobacillus* and bifidobacteria as well as *Streptococcus thermophilus*. Kefir is also a very rich source of nutrients, including vitamin B_{12}, which is hard to find in the vegetable kingdom. (Although not technically a vegetable, vegans generally find drinking kefir that has been cultured in water acceptable.)

Traditionally, kefir grains are added to cow's, goat's or sheep's milk, covered, but not sealed, and then left at room temperature for 24–48 hours until the mixture is slightly fizzy, then the grains are drained, the yoghurt-like drink is drunk, and the grains are added to the next milk drink to repeat the process, and so on.

If you wish to avoid dairy, you can make a kefir drink by adding one teaspoon of sugar to a large glass or container containing 500ml pure water, plus a squeeze of lemon juice and leave to ferment as above. Strain off the kefir grains and drink the kefir water, then start again. It tastes like slightly fizzy, but unsweet, lemonade.

You can also make kefir with fruit juice or coconut milk. The process is the same. Whether you use milk (containing the milk sugar lactose), fruit juice or coconut milk or you just add sugar to water, it needs a source of sugar to multiply. The sugar is used up in the fermenting process, so the end result is a more or less sugar-free drink. If you make your kefir in coconut milk, you will have to put the grains in dairy milk after about 4 times of using in order that the grains can feed and grow. Leave for 24–48 hours as before, then strain and continue with your preferred liquid.

There are over 200 studies already published on kefir[42] showing all kinds of benefits, including a recent study showing that breast cancer cells die off when exposed to kefir.[43] It's certainly a drink to add to a cancer prevention diet. Below are some of the health benefits of kefir found in the studies:

- Enhanced immunity and anti-cancer properties
- Anti-inflammatory effects in the gut
- Anti-microbial effects against *Candida albicans*
- Improved lactose digestion, helping to convert it to lactic acid

Despite containing yeasts, kefir is well tolerated by those with candidiasis, and even helps to kill the bacteria *Candida albicans*. The only hint of a caution I've seen is in one study where mice were infected with *Clostridium difficile* and it made their infection worse, not better. So, if you are battling with *C. difficile*, I'd hold fire on kefir. It is also excellent for stimulating regular bowel movements, hence combating constipation. (See Resources for suppliers of kefir grains as a starter kit.)

Re-inoculating your gut with probiotics

If you have had a major infection or have been treated with antibiotics, you might benefit from a more direct way of 're-inoculating' your digestive tract by taking a probiotic supplement. The more 'broad spectrum' the antibiotic, the more likely it is to devastate your colony of beneficial bacteria, leaving you even more susceptible to infection. Alcohol, in excess, also messes up your microbiota.[44] Taking probiotics with antibiotics more than halves the overgrowth of less desirable microorganisms such as coliforms, enterococci and *Staphylococcus aureus*.[45]

Health-food stores stock probiotic supplements, many of which contain a combination of beneficial bacteria. The two most common families of bacteria provided are *Lactobacillus acidophilus* and bifidobacteria. Different strains are included according to whether the supplements are designed for children or adults, so you should seek advice on the best one to take, depending on your circumstances.

These supplements are made by culturing bacteria, then freeze-drying them. They are quite delicate organisms and are best kept in the fridge. When you swallow them and they come into contact with moisture, they come back to life. The best probiotic supplements also contain FOS for the bacteria to feed off, promoting their rapid multiplication, so check the label. FOS can also be supplemented on its own and has been shown to help promote more of the good bacteria and reduce the bad, as well as relieving constipation.[46]

Generally, you will need to take one or two capsules, or a

teaspoon a day, providing around a billion of each strain of bacteria. It's best to take them with food if the bacteria are micro-encapsulated or enteric coated. Otherwise, take them away from meals to minimise their destruction from the gastric acid in the stomach. If you are taking probiotics therapeutically (for example, to re-inoculate the digestive tract after antibiotics or as part of an anti-infection strategy to kill off candidiasis), you might need three times this amount. These higher levels of probiotics and prebiotics such as FOS do sometimes result in increased flatulence, at least in the short term. This is not necessarily a bad sign. Sometimes, as less desirable organisms die off, symptoms get worse before they get better.

Summary – Chapter 7

Here are a few steps that you can take to promote healthy intestinal flora:

- Eat a more plant-based diet.
- Eat fermented foods such as yoghurt, miso, shoyu, sauerkraut, sourdough bread and kefir.
- Take a probiotic supplement containing beneficial strains of bacteria as well as FOS on a regular basis.
- Limit alcohol and take a probiotic supplement after excessive alcohol intake.
- Take a higher-dose probiotic supplement for 2–4 weeks after a course of antibiotics.
- Consider supplementing probiotics for any of the conditions listed above.

In Part III I'll refer to specific strains and combinations more likely to be effective against specific digestive concerns.

CHAPTER 8

Digestive Irritants – from Alcohol to Antibiotics

Many substances that we consume on a daily basis (quite apart from those foods that we are allergic or intolerant to) are digestive irritants. These include alcohol, antibiotics, painkillers, certain spices, modern wheat, coffee and tea. In excess, these alone can be the cause of digestive problems.

Alcohol

An intestinal irritant, alcohol causes inflammation and damage to the digestive-tract wall, also depleting healthy gut bacteria.[47] This increases the risk of abnormal intestinal permeability, which, in turn, increases the likelihood of an allergic reaction, especially to the ingredients contained in the alcoholic drink. For this reason, about one in five beer and wine drinkers (on testing) show sensitivity to yeast. Wine drinkers become sensitive to sulphites, which are added to grapes to control their fermentation. Sulphites are also found in exhaust fumes; and the liver enzyme that detoxifies sulphites is dependent on molybdenum, a trace element that many people are deficient in. It's better to choose organic, sulphite-free wines and champagnes – and the latter has the added bonus of being yeast-free.

As well as increasing intestinal permeability, alcohol wreaks havoc on intestinal bacteria, encouraging a proliferation of cells in the colon, which can initiate cancer. It can also be absorbed directly into the mucosal cells that line the digestive tract, and converted into aldehyde, which interferes with DNA repair and promotes tumours. In addition, some alcoholic drinks contain the carcinogen urethane. This is formed as a result of a chemical reaction that occurs during fermentation, baking or storage and has been found in American bourbon, European fruit brandies, cream sherries, port, saké and Chinese wine, but not vodka, gin or most beers.

According to the World Health Organisation, drinking alcohol has been linked to cancer of the throat, mouth, larynx, pharynx, oesophagus, bladder, breast and liver, with a substantially higher risk in those who smoke *and* drink. The World Cancer Research Fund reached the same conclusions back in 1997. The evidence has only got stronger since, and points to the fact that the increased risk of colon and breast cancer occurs at very low levels of consumption. In the case of breast cancer a link starts to emerge above four drinks a week, while for colon cancer this association becomes stronger above a drink a day.

Although there is a mildly protective effect from small amounts of red wine in relation to heart disease, overall regular alcohol consumption is very bad news for digestion and increases the risk of cancer. Specifically, it increases the risk of abnormal intestinal permeability and allergies, and is therefore best avoided during any digestive-health programme.

Antibiotics

Antibiotics are designed to kill bacteria, and, as we have seen, the more 'broad spectrum' an antibiotic is, the more it damages the vital, health-promoting bacteria in the digestive tract.

What is more, the large quantity of antibiotic you need to consume to get enough into the bloodstream to fight, for instance, a sinus infection, creates a massive overload of antibiotics, especially in the upper digestive tract. Since the intestinal flora protect the digestive tract, their destruction soon leads to inflammation and discomfort (experienced by most people taking antibiotics within 48 hours).

Antibiotics increase intestinal permeability and the risk and severity of allergies; for example, treating a child with an ear infection with antibiotics increases their risk of having another ear infection by five times.[48] This is because recurrent ear infections, in my clinical experience, are often the consequence of an allergy or food intolerance triggering inflammation, most often to dairy products, which results in excessive mucus production.

With the current global use of over 63,000 tons of antibiotics each year in agriculture, expected to reach over 100,000 tons by 2030, and over 50 billion antibiotic treatments prescribed annually by doctors, animals – including us – are becoming less resistant to disease, and bacteria are becoming more resistant to antibiotics. There is little doubt that this has played a part in the rapid escalation of food poisoning, which now kills more than a million people a year worldwide. In the US alone the US Centers for Disease

Control and Prevention (CDC) estimates that antibiotic resistance is responsible for more than 2 million infections and 23,000 deaths.[49] For more on antibiotics see Chapter 13.

Painkillers

The most commonly used painkillers, known as nonsteroidal anti-inflammatory drugs (NSAIDs), are very bad news for digestion. These include ibuprofen (Motrin), fenoprofen (Fenopron), flurbiprofen (Froben), ketoprofen (Alrheumat, Orudis and Oruvail), naproxen (Naprosyn), tolmetin (Tolectin), sulindac (Clinoril), azapropazone (Rheumox), indomethacin (Indocid), phenylbutazone (Butazolidine), mefenamic acid (Ponstan), diclofenac (Voltarol), fenbufen (Lederfen), piroxicam (Feldene), tiaprofenic acid (Surgam), as well as aspirin. (See Chapter 13 for more about NSAIDs.) In England alone, around 68 million painkiller prescriptions are written each year, many of which are for NSAIDs, which is only a fraction of the amount bought over the counter. The average person takes 373 painkillers a year.[50] The first drug that tends to be used to relieve pain and inflammation is aspirin; it can be quite effective but is hard on the digestion. As far back as 1980, the sixth World Nutrition Congress reported that even a single aspirin can cause intestinal bleeding for one week. Just imagine what high doses on a daily basis over many years are likely to do. NSAIDs increase gut permeability[51] and ulcers in the small intestine, which can lead to serious complications. A study of athletes at the University of Iowa in the US, who took aspirin in order to prevent any inflammation, found that it significantly increased their intestinal permeability.[52] NSAIDS are also known to increase indigestion.[53]A significant proportion of ulcers in the small intestine might be due to these drugs.[54] At least nine NSAIDs have been withdrawn from use, and they are responsible for one-quarter of all the reported adverse medication reactions. In the US, the nation's spending on NSAIDs roughly equals the cost of treating the side effects, many of which are gastro-intestinal reactions.

Paracetamol doesn't have the same irritant effect as NSAIDs, but it is bad news for the liver. Gastrointestinal irritation from painkillers overloads the liver's ability to detoxify (explained in Chapter 27), which is further compromised through use of this painkilling drug. For more on painkillers and the new class of anti-inflammatory drugs that don't damage the gut but do have other side effects, read Chapter 13.

Coffee and tea

Coffee contains a group of substances known as methylxan-thines, that include caffeine, theobromine and theophylline. These irritate the digestive tract and also bind to minerals, removing them before they are absorbed. The consequences of drinking too much coffee, therefore, are gastrointestinal irritation, reflux and poor absorption of nutrients. Some people are more sensitive than others. The same is true to an extent for tea, although the chemicals present are somewhat different: tea has less caffeine but more tannin, which binds to minerals and escorts them out of the body.

The odd cup of tea or coffee is unlikely to be a problem; however, anyone who is experiencing digestive problems, and has a regular or excessive intake of tea or coffee, is well advised to quit during a digestive-healing programme.

Although herb and fruit teas don't contain gut irritants,

any very hot drink is stressful on the digestive tract. The incidence of oesophageal cancer and stomach problems is higher among those who consume very hot drinks on a regular basis, so, it's best to avoid scaldingly hot drinks.

Spices

Not all spices are created equal as far as digestion is concerned. Top of the 'bad' list is chilli, at least for some. This acts as an intestinal irritant, especially in large amounts, and many people are actually quite allergic to it. If you don't react well to very spicy-hot foods, it is quite likely that you are allergic or sensitive to chilli.

There are, however, other spices that don't irritate the digestive tract and might even be beneficial. These include cayenne pepper, which contains capsaicin, a known anti-inflammatory agent. Capsaicin has been shown in many studies to reduce inflammation effectively. It also stimulates saliva production – potentially good for those suffering from a dry mouth.[55]

Curcumin is the bright yellow pigment of the spice turmeric and has a variety of powerful anti-inflammatory effects; thus it is good for the digestive tract. Curcumin has also been shown to promote detoxification, helping to detoxify, among other substances, alcohol.

Fibre and ileo-caecal valve problems

Although eating an unrefined diet, high in fibre, is generally good for you, some people experience a problem with certain kinds of fibre such as bran, and even raw foods. If this is true for you and you have inconsistent bowel movements – perhaps sometimes with diarrhoea and at other times constipation – you might have a problem with your ileo-caecal valve. This is a circular valve-like muscle that separates the small intestine from the large intestine. It is located almost exactly midway between the right hip bone and tummy button. If this area is tender when you apply pressure to it, this is a further indication that you might have an inflamed ileo-caecal valve.

If the ileo-caecal valve doesn't open and close properly, or is too open, bacteria and toxins from the large intestine can move more easily than they should into the small intestine, leading to bacterial imbalance and self-intoxication. Proper ileo-caecal function can be disrupted by a diet that is too high in digestive irritants, including coarse fibres, or by constipation or the loss of proper muscle tone and peristaltic muscle action that moves faecal matter along.

In such cases, the ileo-caecal valve function can be restored by two methods. One is a physical technique of manipulation practised by naturopaths, some nutritionists and kinesiologists. The other is by eating a diet that is very low in digestive irritants for a couple of weeks. This means excluding all the foods and drinks discussed in this chapter as well as wheat bran and any raw foods. Rather than adding fibre, or eating foods with added wheat fibre, which is very coarse, it is much better to obtain your fibre from whole foods and, where applicable, soak them; for example, if you soak oat flakes to allow them to expand and absorb liquid, the fibres are much gentler on the digestive tract. Similarly, while raw food is good for almost everyone almost all the time, steaming or lightly cooking vegetables partially breaks down the coarser fibres.

Summary – Chapter 8

If you want to be kind to your digestive tract:

- Avoid a regular intake of tea, coffee and alcohol.
- Minimise your use of painkilling drugs, especially NSAIDs.
- Only consider antibiotics as a last resort, and, after a course of antibiotics, always take probiotics to restore your intestinal flora.
- Don't eat food spiced with chilli on a regular basis.
- Avoid added wheat bran – eat whole, unrefined foods instead.

CHAPTER 9

Our Deadly Bread

Conventional healthy-eating advice is that wheat and whole grains should be a major part of our diet and that a small fraction of people, perhaps one in three thousand, are intolerant to a protein in wheat called gluten and suffer with celiac disease. (In the UK the spelling is 'coeliac' but I'll use 'celiac' as this is more prevalent globally.) Every part of that opening sentence is wrong, and I'd like to explain why. Firstly, the wheat you eat today bears little resemblance to the wheat mankind has eaten for thousands of years. Not surprisingly, for reasons that will become clear, many of us do badly on this food, with varying degrees of intolerance. Secondly, it is now clear that celiac disease, which can be fatal, is much more common than previously thought, and is on the increase, affecting as many as one in a hundred people.

Celiac disease – a growing problem

A variety of health problems, including slow growth as a child and fatigue as an adult, can be caused by celiac disease. A study involving 5,000 high-school students in central Italy found that the prevalence of celiac disease was close to one in every 200 students, with five in every six cases undiagnosed.[56] One study shows that eight out of ten celiac sufferers, chronically allergic to gliadin, go undiagnosed.[57] Some countries are more aware of the problem than others. In Finland 25 per cent of celiacs are diagnosed by their doctor. In Italy only 6 per cent are diagnosed.[58] Celiac disease is thought to be such a health threat in Italy that the government has considered mandating that all children, regardless of whether they are sick or not, must be tested for gliadin sensitivity and celiac disease by 6 years of age. In the United Kingdom we are still in the Dark Ages in terms of recognising the widespread prevalence of celiac disease.

Celiac disease leads to severe malabsorption of nutrients, which can result in serious complications in later life, such as infertility, psychiatric disorders, osteoporosis and cancer. The condition does not always present with classical symptoms (including iron-deficiency anaemia, as well as short stature, mentioned earlier), which leaves many sufferers undiagnosed. It is vastly underdiagnosed, with correct diagnosis taking on average 11 years! The first manifesting symptoms are not uncommonly depression (not all sufferers originally report gut problems) or gastrointestinal cancer, by which time it is often too late. Of those with digestive problems, about one in 40 children and one in 30 adults have celiac disease, although few are diagnosed as such.[59]

The symptoms of wheat gluten sensitivity

You don't have to have celiac disease to be sensitive to wheat. At last the medical profession is starting to acknowledge the existence of 'non-celiac gluten sensitivity'. The most common symptoms of wheat sensitivity are constipation, diarrhoea, abdominal bloating or pain; however, many other symptoms have also been reported in those found to be sensitive to wheat. These include:

acne and boils
anxiety and paranoia
apathy and confusion
cramps
depression
fatigue
flatulence
migraine
nausea
skin rashes
sweating
throat trouble

If you suffer from any of the above, you should take the possibility of wheat intolerance seriously. This might affect between one in five and one in ten people (10–20 per cent). Twenty years ago, at the Institute for Optimum Nutrition, my colleagues and I ran a small study investigating the effects of removing wheat from the diet of 66 people who had digestive problems. They all craved bread and, as a result, ate a lot of it, not realising that wheat might be causing their digestive problems. During the study they abstained from eating wheat for a period of six weeks to investigate the possibility of a food allergy or intolerance. A total of 90 per cent experienced improvements in all their digestive symptoms, and 6 per cent had between 75 and 100 per cent improvement in all their symptoms. Six symptoms were reduced dramatically: constipation, flatulence, bloating, food cravings, lack of energy and mood swings. It is reasonable to suggest that these subjects were suffering from wheat intolerance.[60]

Although many so-called experts have often dismissed these apparent signs of wheat intolerance, recent research has found distinct evidence that non-celiacs with wheat sensitivity actually do have immune reactions to wheat, with increased antibodies against wheat in their gut and bloodstream. Both types of antibodies were found: IgE (for allergies) and IgG (for intolerances).[61] (See Chapter 10 for more on these.) (See Resources for a home test kit for both IgG antibody sensitivity and celiac disease.)

One very likely reason for this ever-growing problem, which I estimate affects at least one in ten people, is that the wheat we eat today, which in some products has a higher glycemic index (GI) than white sugar, bears little resemblance to the wheat mankind has eaten for thousands of years. Modern wheat has a higher concentration of gluten. This is because a high level of gluten makes a lighter loaf. When yeast is fed sugar it produces gas, and in the presence of the sticky protein gluten this makes bubbles, and hence lighter loaves. Baked products then look bigger and sell better. This kind of baking increases the amount of gluten available to react with the gut wall. So although high-gluten wheat might be good for the baking industry, it's bad for your digestion.

The history of wheat

One of the first wheat varieties our ancestors ate, going back to 3300BC, was called einkorn. It's in a very simple category of wheat, genetically speaking. Shortly after it began to be cultivated, it crossed with goat grass, giving rise to a more complex wheat category called tetraploid. In this category we find durum (normally used for pasta) and the ancient grains, known as emmer and khorasan (*Triticum turgidum*) wheat, now sold under the trademark of Kamut Khorosan®. That is what mankind basically ate for the next few thousand years; for example, einkorn has been found in pharaohs' tombs whereas emmer and khorasan were eaten by ancient civilisations in Mesopotamia.

The ancient Kamut khorasan is the only wheat I like to eat and it comes down to us unchanged from ancient times. (The Kamut trademark is a guarantee that this wheat is an unchanged ancient grain and also exclusively grown organically in much the same way it would have been cultivated thousands of years ago. Also, it has to have a guaranteed minimum level of various essential elements, effectively guaranteeing that it is grown in good soil.)

At some point tetraploid wheat crossed with a grass called *Triticum tauschii* to form *Triticum aestivum*, a category of wheat known as hexaploid. Examples of wheat grown today in this group are spelt, and its close cousin *T. vulgare*, which is common bread wheat; however, the original bread wheat is fundamentally different from the modern bread wheat you are likely to eat today. Modern wheat has undergone thousands of hybridisations to increase yield (making the wheat plentiful and cheap), and also to increase and change the quality of the gluten content, which, as we have seen, enables the loaf to rise to a larger size. However, it seems to be the *qualitative* difference in gliadin, rather than the quantity, that is the problem. This explains why today's wheat has many more gluten proteins than were ever present in original wheat strains. In one hybridisation experiment, 14 new gluten proteins were identified.[62]

Imagine the chemical difference between modern and ancient wheat now that today's wheat has been through thousands of hybridisations. It has been extremely modified or changed for reasons of profit rather than health. This madness is now continuing at a new level as biotech companies strive to create and then introduce strains of GMO wheat that can be patented and is compatible with specific pesticides and chemical treatments. The net result, even before GMO wheat is perfected and introduced, is that the gluten proteins in today's wheat are substantially different from the gluten proteins, as well as other compounds, found in the earliest forms of wheat, such as Kamut khorasan.

The problems with gliadins and glutenins

The two main families of gluten proteins are called 'gliadins' and 'glutenins'. Oats, for example, contain no gliadins and, probably consequently, are a much less allergenic food. Gliadin is now recognised as the offending gluten, so oats are now considered gluten-free, unless contaminated with wheat in storage or production. Old wheats tend to have fewer, and different, gliadins.[63] A particular form of gliadin, called alpha-gliadin, inflames the intestine, causing abdominal cramps and diarrhoea. Gliadin is particularly tricky because it has a unique ability to get through the intestinal wall. It triggers the release of a protein called zonulin (explained on page 42), which literally opens up gaps between the intestinal cells, increasing gastrointestinal permeability. This, in turn, means that whole food proteins can cross the gut barrier, triggering the immune system to react, which is the basis for developing food intolerances. It also damages the villi in the gut wall. When rats are fed modern wheat these villi atrophy, but this doesn't happen with Kamut khorasan.[64] Old strains of wheat also trigger less inflammation than modern wheat.[65]

Thorough food intolerance testing laboratories measure the presence of not only IgG antibodies to a wide variety of foods, which means your system has become sensitised, but also to gliadin itself. If you are diagnosed as gliadin sensitive it is well worth avoiding wheat for at least three months.

Durum wheat (at least the original form, now itself hybridised beyond recognition) is used to make pasta. It is also a genetically simpler form of wheat (tetraploid), although I prefer to eat Kamut pasta.

Pasta has a fraction of the GI or GL of wheat bread, which raises your blood sugar levels, and hence insulin, quite dramatically. The increased insulin and blood sugar levels feed into abdominal weight gain and, ultimately, diabetes.

Wheat messes with your mind – and your middle

I have long known that wheat intolerance can be the cause of schizophrenia symptoms through working with many diagnosed schizophrenics who had, in some cases, complete relief through wheat avoidance. I remember the case of one young woman, Erica, whom I met in her early twenties, who had suffered for years from schizophrenia. She had dropped out of school, but she went on to get a degree, marry, and raise a family after excluding wheat from her diet.

I had become aware of this link through the research of Curtis Dohan, a psychiatrist, who reported relief of schizophrenia symptoms when he removed wheat from his diet. This was published in the *British Medical Journal* back in the 1970s when I was studying psychology. Wheat can also exacerbate symptoms of ADHD (attention deficit hyperactivity disorder) and autism.

This link with mental-health problems led to the discovery that modern wheat, during its digestion, generates peptides (combinations of amino acids) that mimic opioids (heroin and morphine are opioids) called gluteomorphins, which occupy the same receptors in the brain as heroin.[66] Gluteomorphins are commonly found in the urine of children diagnosed with autism.

The effect of these gluteomorphins, created when you digest modern wheat, is that you want more. Wheat literally becomes addictive. Combined with the sugar load created by yeast-activated bakery products, and the subsequent blood sugar low, which stimulates appetite, modern wheat is literally an appetite stimulant. This is, of course, great news for the food industry and one of the reasons why wheat-eating nations have a big problem with ever-increasing belly fat.

I have had so many clients who have reported massive weight loss, and a cessation of abdominal bloating, by excluding modern wheat. There's a very good book, *Wheat Belly* by William Davis, that argues why our modern-day obsession with wheat is driving abdominal weight gain, although he fails to differentiate between the effects of modern wheat and ancient wheats that are available today, such as Kamut khorasan.

Wheat promotes inflammation

When you gain abdominal fat, known as visceral fat, it triggers part of the body's inflammatory response mechanism. This, in turn, makes you both more likely to become intolerant or allergic and to develop inflammatory symptoms, the classics being headaches, eczema or dermatitis, asthma, irritable bowel diseases such as Crohn's and ulcerative colitis, rhinitis, arthritis – and just about any other '-itis'.

Although the general view is that gluten is the culprit, I am beginning to revise this simplistic opinion after a series of experiments that have been carried out on Kamut khorasan wheat.[67] Technically, Kamut *does* contain gluten proteins and, as such, should promote inflammation; however, it doesn't. A series of well-conducted studies have shown that Kamut grain is not only anti-inflammatory but it also has a powerful antioxidant effect. In addition, although regular wheat causes atrophy (damage) to the villi in the digestive tract, the Kamut does not.

That's all well and good in lab studies, but what happens in real life when humans eat this grain?

Ancient Kamut brand wheat is anti-inflammatory

A randomised double-blind study was published on people with irritable bowel syndrome (IBS), carried out by researchers at the University of Florence in Italy.[68] The participants were given foods (bread, pasta, biscuits and crackers) made from either modern wheat or Kamut wheat. They didn't know which kind of food they were eating and they were randomly assigned to eating either modern wheat products or Kamut products for six weeks at a time. Then, after a break for six weeks, the type of wheat they were eating was switched and they continued to eat the new diet for another six weeks. Their symptoms of IBS were meticulously recorded.

During the modern-wheat weeks they had no improvement, and continued to suffer from abdominal pain, bloating, tiredness and irregular and unhealthy bowel movements. However, when they were unknowingly eating Kamut, everything got better. They reported significantly less bloating, abdominal pain, irregularity and tiredness, with a much higher overall measure of quality of life.

Also, convincingly, markers of inflammation in the blood, known as pro-inflammatory cytokines, which are usually raised in people with IBS, all reduced. This is exactly the opposite of what one would expect with conventional wheat that is high in gluten proteins. This effect, as seen in blood markers, has been found in every human trial using Kamut khorasan, including in people with cardiovascular disease, diabetes and fatty liver disease.[69]

I am starting to think that the main problem with wheat is not gluten or gliadin per se, but the fact that we are eating a food that is considerably different genetically and chemically to that which we may have become adapted to eat in reasonable quantities. The solution for wheat-intolerant people might not always be strict avoidance of wheat and other gluten or gliadin grains, but rather the avoidance of *modern* wheat.

Gluten is present in wheat, rye, barley and oats, although, as we have seen, oats contain no gliadin. Spelt is probably a less adulterated form of modern wheat, but it is quite different and genetically much more complex that the original ancient grain, such as Kamut. Spelt is a hexaploid wheat, as is modern wheat.

Kamut is higher than modern wheat in antioxidants and polyphenols, which are generally anti-inflammatory, as well as magnesium, potassium, selenium, iron, zinc and other important minerals. Unlike spelt, Kamut is *only* grown organically, with no exposure to modern chemicals, in other words in conditions that most closely resemble those we may have adapted to over the thousands of years of wheat consumption, from the early days when mankind moved from hunter-gatherer to peasant farmer.

Kamut is fast becoming a fashionable superfood in the US, where it is grown (it is primarily grown in Montana and its neighbouring states for the North American market where 80,000 acres are now under organic cultivation). It is also well known and popular in Italy and gradually becoming available in the UK. (See Resources for a list of the range of Kamut products now available in the UK.)

Gluten-free grains

Although it is clear that many people react differently to ancient wheat than to modern wheat, for those with celiac disease it is wise to avoid all gluten-containing grains and choose gluten-free grains instead, as shown below:

Gluten-containing grains	Gluten-free grains
Wheat	Corn (maize)
Rye	Rice
Spelt	Oats
Barley	Buckwheat
	Gram (chickpea flour)
	Quinoa

Often, as part of a digestive-healing programme, it is wise to go on a no-wheat, low-gluten diet for a month. Fortunately, there are many wheat-free and gluten-free options to choose from in health-food shops and supermarkets these days:

- **Breads** Cornbread, rice cakes, oatcakes
- **Pasta** Buckwheat spaghetti, soba noodles

(buckwheat), rice noodles, quinoa pasta, corn pasta, polenta (cornmeal)

- **Cereals** Cornflakes, oatmeal, rice cereal, millet flakes

If you do not have celiac disease, however, it is well worth experimenting with Kamut khorasan breads, pastas and bulgar. I have not seen any negative effects, only positive, in all the studies on ancient Kamut khorasan wheat and have met many people who are sensitive to wheat who have noticed a clear improvement, such as Mary below.

Case Study: Mary

Mary had suffered with bloating, wind and urgent trips to the loo for the previous four years – these are classic signs of IBS – seemingly after eating wheat.

'I assumed it was gluten intolerance, but it wasn't because I even reacted to some gluten-free flours, especially cornflour. I also react to spelt, but when I started eating Kamut khorasan wheat, to my amazement, I had absolutely no problem. I can eat a whole loaf of Kamut khorasan bread in a day (!) and not suffer any ill health at all.

'Having used Kamut khorasan products for five months now, my health has returned and I feel alive once more. Last week I ate some regular bread and reacted immediately. I make my own Kamut khorasan bread, which is delicious, and it's the best flour I've ever used for bread and other products. It tastes as if it is doing you good and, in my case, it clearly is.'

Summary – Chapter 9

Generally speaking, to avoid the problems discussed in this chapter:

- Don't eat wheat every day; choose gluten-free, Kamut khorasan or low-gluten grains instead. Also choose wholegrain.
- When you eat breads, choose heavier, lower-gluten breads.
- Vary the grains you eat – have rye, oats, rice, barley, buckwheat, quinoa, corn.
- Limit grains to no more than a quarter of your total dietary intake.
- If you have a digestive problem or inflammatory bowel problem, investigate whether you are wheat- or gluten-sensitive with an IgG food intolerance test and a celiac test to measure IgATT (see Resources).

CHAPTER 10

Food Allergies, Intolerances and Sensitivities

Very much on the increase, food allergies and intolerances are an almost inevitable consequence of problems with digestion and absorption. An estimated one in three people has an allergy or intolerance. Some of these are to airborne substances such as pollen (hay fever), house dust mites or cat's fur; others are to chemicals in food, household products or the environment. But the most common category of allergy- and intolerance-provoking substances is the food we eat. In a survey of 3,300 adults, 43 per cent said they experienced adverse reactions to food.[70]

The illustration overleaf shows the variety of symptoms associated with allergies or intolerances. If you have three or more of these symptoms, you probably have an allergy, intolerance or sensitivity, and it will most likely be related to something you are eating.

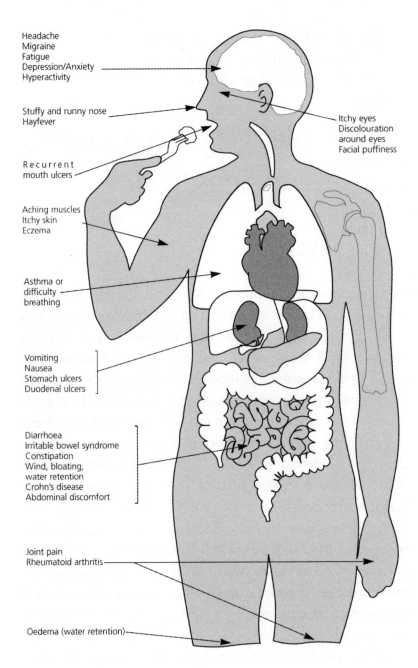

Headache
Migraine
Fatigue
Depression/Anxiety
Hyperactivity

Stuffy and runny nose
Hayfever

Recurrent
mouth ulcers

Aching muscles
Itchy skin
Eczema

Asthma or
difficulty
breathing

Vomiting
Nausea
Stomach ulcers
Duodenal ulcers

Diarrhoea
Irritable bowel syndrome
Constipation
Wind, bloating,
water retention
Crohn's disease
Abdominal discomfort

Joint pain
Rheumatoid arthritis

Oedema (water retention)

Itchy eyes
Discolouration
around eyes
Facial puffiness

Symptoms associated with food allergy and intolerance

The most common allergy/intolerance-provoking foods are:

wheat (bread, biscuits, cereals, pasta)
dairy produce (milk, cheese, yoghurt)
alcohol (especially beer and wine)
yeast
coffee
tea
chocolate
nuts
eggs
oranges
chemical additives in food

If you eat any one of these foods two or three times a day and would find them difficult to give up, it might be worth being tested to see if you're intolerant to them, or any other foods that you eat. This happens because the gut's immune system GALT (gut-associated lymphatic system) is highly active and behaves like a bouncer at the gateway to your body. If foods arrive at the gate undigested, or if the gate is damaged and inflamed, the ensuing chaos usually leads to some 'arrests' by the immune police. This triggers an allergic and/or inflammatory reaction experienced as swelling and pain, which might not be localised to the gut. This is, in essence, what most food allergies or intolerances are all about. Of course, the real solution to food intolerances is to heal the digestive system and eat foods that don't stress or irritate the digestive tract; however, if you've already developed intolerances, you first need to 'undevelop' them by finding out which foods you are currently reacting to and avoiding them for a long enough period in which to heal the digestive tract and reprogram the immune police.

Before we explore how to do this, it's important to clarify the difference between a food allergy, a food intolerance and an enzyme deficiency; for example, many people who can't digest lactose, the sugar in milk, believe that they have a milk allergy. A milk allergy is an allergic reaction to the *protein* in milk, and is actually quite rare. I have this. What most people have is an enzyme deficiency called lactose intolerance, which means that they are intolerant to the *sugar* in milk; an IgG-mediated milk intolerance is quite common. IgG is an antibody that shows up in tests when you have a food intolerance; I'll explain this in detail later in the chapter.

Common causes of gut sensitivities

If you are suffering from bloating, belching, indigestion, heartburn, abdominal pain, IBS or any other digestive complaint, or if you have other symptoms after meals, you might be wondering if there's something you are eating that you are intolerant or allergic to.

Actually, they are not the only things that can cause sensitivities to certain foods, and you can find out what's going on with a few simple experiments. Each day, your body produces 10 litres of digestive juices containing enzymes, acids and other secretions that break down food. There are different enzymes and secretions for different foods; for example, protein needs stomach acid, then a sequence of protein-splitting enzymes such as pepsin, protease, and so on. Fat, on the other hand, needs lipase and bile, made in the liver. Milk needs lactase. Greens need glucosidase whereas beans need galactosidase, as do cruciferous veg such as broccoli.

The first test, especially if your symptoms include bloating and indigestion straight after certain meals, is to take a digestive enzyme supplement containing all the above. If the problem goes away, you know that your problem is your body is not producing enough of the right enzymes for certain food groups (see Chapter 2). Knowing this, you'll be able to work out by trial and error which foods are difficult for you.

The reason for the bloating is that if you don't digest foods completely, bacteria in your gut will feed on it and produce gas.

Some people, especially later in life, don't make enough stomach acid and can suffer with indigestion, bloating and, ironically, heartburn. The heartburn is caused by very small amounts of stomach acid getting through the shut-off valve at the top of the stomach and into the oesophagus leading to the throat. Without sufficient stomach acid, food can't be properly digested and harmful bacteria will not be killed off. The correct balance of bacteria in the gut therefore becomes disrupted. The net result can be more upward gas, leading to belching, and heartburn caused by acid leaking. If a person underproduces stomach acid, this can be supplemented as betaine hydrochloride. I explain how to do this in Chapter 17.

This then points towards the next test. You might have an imbalance of the correct bacteria in the gut – this is called dysbiosis. Although there are stool tests (available through nutritional therapists) that can measure what's going on, I often recommend two weeks to a month of taking a good probiotic supplement a day. This needs to contain both *Lactobacillus acidophilus* and bifidobacteria, and at least 1–5 billion viable organisms per dose. If this solves your problem, all well and good, but there are some gut issues that need a different approach. An example of this is infection with *Helicobacter pylori*, the organism that causes most stomach ulcers, as described on page 32 (more on this in Chapter 18).

Another example would be some kind of food poisoning, in which case you might need antibiotics if it doesn't resolve quickly. If you experience a sudden onset of symptoms, perhaps vomiting or diarrhoea, food poisoning is the likely culprit.

I recommend taking probiotics to restore healthy gut bacteria after taking antibiotics.

Food allergy or intolerance?

If you've ruled out indigestion and dysbiosis, the next most likely contributor to your digestive problems would be a food allergy or intolerance.

The classic definition of an allergy is 'any idiosyncratic reaction where the immune system is clearly involved'. The immune system (the body's defence system) can produce 'markers' for substances it doesn't like. The classic markers are antibodies called IgE (immunoglobulin type E). These attach themselves to 'mast cells' in the body. When the offending food (or allergen) combines with its specific IgE antibody, the IgE molecule triggers the mast cell to release granules containing histamine and other chemicals that cause the typical symptoms of allergy: skin rashes, hay fever, rhinitis, sinusitis, asthma and eczema. Severe allergies to shellfish or peanuts, for example, can cause immediate gastrointestinal upsets or swelling in the face or throat. All these reactions are immediate, severe and inflammatory. They are known as type-1 allergic reactions and you are likely to know you have them. However, other people suffer from chronic conditions, and they are always eating an offending food, but it can take decades, if ever, to make the link between the two.

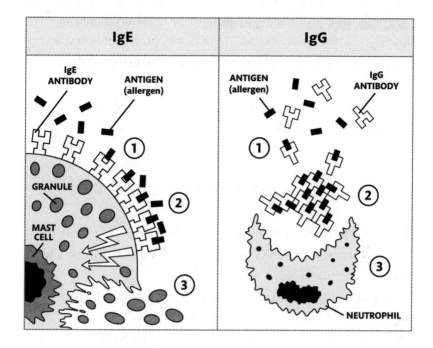

How IgG and IgE reactions happen

Testing for these allergies involves a pin prick containing a drop of potential allergens; if you react, you get a red wheal. This immediate reaction, which occurs within ten minutes, is an IgE reaction.

The most common reactions – IgG

Many reactions against food involve a different kind of antibody, however, called IgG. Most people call these 'food intolerances', in order to distinguish them from the potentially life-threatening effects of classical IgE allergy reactions, even though they do fit the bill for the definition of an allergic reaction. IgG reactions don't occur immediately, so it isn't always easy to know what you are reacting to.

Food Reaction	% Population	Test(s) Required
True allergy	Approx. 2% (adults)	Blood test for food-specific IgE antibodies
Celiac disease	Approx. 1% (varies from country to country)	Blood tests for anti-endomysial and anti-transglutaminase antibodies, and total IgA antibodies
Lactose intolerance	5% Northern Europe (higher in Southern Europe, Asia, Africa)	Hydrogen breath test
IgG-mediated food intolerance	Approx. 45%	Finger-prick blood test for food-specific IgG antibodies

Dr James Braly, former director of Immuno Laboratories, which developed the IgG ELISA test, now the gold standard for food-intolerance testing, says, 'Food intolerance is not rare, nor are the effects limited to the air passages, the skin and digestive tract. Most food intolerances are delayed reactions, taking anywhere from an hour to three days to show themselves, and are therefore much harder to detect. Delayed food intolerance appears to be simply the inability of your digestive tract to prevent large quantities of partially digested and undigested food from entering the bloodstream.'

This is not a new idea. Since the 1950s, pioneering allergists (such as Dr Theron Randolph, Dr William Philpott and Dr Marshall Mandel) have written about delayed sensitivities having far-reaching effects on all systems of the body. These used to be the 'heretics' of classic allergy theory. But now their theories are being proved right, as scientific methods are developed for determining other types of immune reaction. IgG antibodies were first discovered in the 1960s and, despite hundreds of research trials, are still considered rather irrelevant by some conventional medics. The problem, say the critics, is that most people have many IgG-based reactions to foods without apparently suffering from food intolerance reactions. The theory is that IgG antibodies might serve as 'tags' but they don't initiate a reaction; however, say the advocates, a large build-up of IgG antibodies to a particular food indicates a chronic, long-term sensitivity, or food intolerance.

According to Dr Jonathan Brostoff, consultant in medical immunology at the Middlesex Hospital Medical School, certain ingested substances can cause the release of histamine and provoke classic allergic symptoms without involving IgE. These include lectins (in peanuts), shellfish, tomatoes, pork, alcohol, chocolate, pineapple, papaya, buckwheat, sunflower, mango and mustard. He also thinks it is possible that undigested proteins could directly affect mast cells (which, as we have seen, contain histamine) in the gut, causing the classic symptoms of food intolerance. Mast-cell activation can be triggered by many factors, both immune and non-immune, including gut-flora imbalance and factors linked to psychological stress. On activation, mast cells have been linked to chronic pain, inflammation, disturbed gut motility and gut permeability (leaky gut).[71]

One common cause of food intolerance reactions is a substantial production of antibodies (mainly IgG) in response to specific foods in the blood. This results in large immune complexes made by lots of antibodies attaching to the offending food particle. 'It is the sheer weight of numbers that causes a problem,' says Brostoff. 'These immune complexes are like litter going round in the bloodstream.' The litter is cleaned up by cells, principally neutrophils, that act like vacuum cleaners. All this takes time and puts your immune system on red alert, which is what triggers inflammation, the underlying cause of food intolerance symptoms.

These IgG food intolerances are not the same thing as a classic allergy, which is mediated by IgE antibody sensitivity and causes a more immediate reaction by the body's immune system, even to tiny amounts of the allergen.

Evidence of relief through dietary changes

In the last decade, many clinical trials have been published showing that people who avoid the foods they test IgG-intolerant to have a substantial improvement in symptoms. These include studies of those with IBS,[72] inflammatory bowel disease,[73] migraines,[74] weight gain and overall quality of life.[75] In one survey of over 5,000 people who had taken an IgG food intolerance test and avoided their suspect foods, more than three out of four reported a noticeable improvement in their condition, with 68 per cent feeling a benefit within three weeks of following the diet. Of those who rigorously followed the diet, 76 per cent showed noticeable improvement in their chronic symptoms. For those with psychological symptoms, the response rate was 81 per cent, whereas for those with gastrointestinal complaints, such as IBS, the response rate was 80 per cent. For those with depression, 92 per cent responded, and for those with panic attacks all (15 people) benefited. A percentage of 92.3 felt a return of symptoms on reintroduction of the offending foods within the first three months of changing their diet, showing that the correct foods had been identified using this test.[76]

For this reason it is worth having a test to find out what you might be reacting to. This can be done using a tiny amount of blood, collectable with a home test kit. (See Resources to find laboratories carrying out this test.) Once you have the results of your test you will know how strongly your immune system is reacting against certain foods, so you will know which foods to eliminate.

Why might you have a food allergy or intolerance?

Have you ever wondered whether the food you eat actually wants to be eaten? In many cases it appears that it does not. Most foods try their best to protect themselves from predators – with spikes, thorns and chemical toxins.

The idea that food is 'good' is far from accurate. Most foods contain numerous toxins, as well as beneficial nutrients. Omnivores like us have a high-risk–high-return strategy as far as food is concerned. We try different foods, and if we don't get sick, they're OK. But this short-term test can be dangerous. Indeed, even today, the average diet kills most people in the long run.

Some foods are designed to be eaten; for example, many fruits rely on animals eating them to spread the growth of their species. The idea is that animals, such as human beings, eat the fruit and deposit the seed some distance from the original tree with a rich manure starter kit; however, the fruit has to protect itself from unwanted scavengers such as bacteria or fungi that would simply rot the seed. Seeds are therefore often hard to crack and toxic, such as apricot kernels, which contain cyanide compounds. For these reasons, wild food contains a massive and often selective chemical arsenal to ward off specific foes. Food and humans have been fighting for survival since the beginning of time.

Why, then, do food intolerances occur? Are they simply a reaction to less desirable toxins in our food? It is unlikely to be that simple. After all, we too have evolved over millions of years to protect ourselves from chemical poisons with complex detoxification processes that occur mainly in the liver. A number of theories exist, many of which have good supporting evidence.

Could leaky gut syndrome be the problem?

The best place to start our investigation is the digestive tract, since that is where food comes into contact with the body. The textbooks tell us that large food molecules get broken down into simple amino acids, fatty acids and simple sugars. Only these can get into the body. Anything larger is considered a foe. Could it be, however, that undigested food, or leaky gut walls, could expose the immune system to food particles which then trigger a reaction?

This might explain why frequently eaten foods are more likely to cause a reaction. Indeed, recent research shows that people with a food intolerance do tend to have leaky gut walls (explained in detail in Chapter 15). Many food intolerance sufferers may have excessively leaky gut walls, allowing undigested proteins to enter the blood and cause reactions such as the IgG reaction. Consumption of alcohol, the frequent use of aspirin, a deficiency in essential fats or a gastrointestinal infection or infestation (such as candidiasis) are all possible contributors to leaky gut syndrome. All these factors need to be corrected in order to reduce a person's sensitivity to foods. A lack of key nutrients, such as zinc, can also lead to weakening of the gut wall. Of course, poor digestion and a lack of digestive enzymes mean that there are more incompletely digested food proteins available to absorb through a leaky gut.

Gut-associated immune reactions

Although leaky gut syndrome might be part of the reason, it is unlikely to be the whole story. Evidence is accumulating to suggest that the gut wall is far less selective than originally thought, even in healthy people. In one study, healthy adults were given water containing potato starch, which should not normally pass across the gut wall intact. After 15–30 minutes, blood samples contained up to 300 starch grains per millilitre of blood. So why aren't these people developing intolerances? Special immune cells (known as Peyer's patches), which are present in areas along the digestive tract, might provide an explanation. These cells sample the food you eat and desensitise your immune system so that it doesn't react to the food. It seems that most food molecules are recognisably different from undesirable pathogens. Perhaps some people's gut-associated immune system isn't desensitising them to the food they eat.

Indeed, their immune system might even be on red alert when certain food particles arrive. The result of this is that as antibodies are released they attach to the allergen-forming immune complexes and encourage inflammation. As well as leading to symptoms such as bloating, abdominal pain and diarrhoea, this might lead to undigested food passing through the gut wall, causing immune (IgG) reactions in the bloodstream, which then trigger symptoms such as low energy, low mood, migraines, headaches, skin symptoms, joint pains and weight gain, which aren't specifically related to digestion.

Cross-reactions

Another contributor to food sensitivity is exposure to inhalants or other environmental factors that provoke a reaction; for example, it is well known that when the pollen count is high more people suffer from hay fever in polluted areas than in rural areas, despite the lower pollen counts in cities. It is thought that this is because exposure to exhaust fumes makes a pollen-allergic person more sensitive. Whether this is simply because their immune system is weakened from dealing with the pollution, and therefore less able to cope with the additional pollen insult, or due to some kind of cross-reaction, is not known. In the US, where ragweed sensitivity is common, a cross-reaction with bananas has been reported. In other words, one sensitivity sensitises a person to another sensitivity. My theory is that a similar cross-reaction might occur with pollen, wheat and milk for hay-fever sufferers. In practice, avoiding wheat and milk does seem to dramatically relieve hay fever, but this theory has yet to be put to the test.

The emerging view, shared by an increasing number of allergy specialists, is that food sensitivity is a multi-factorial phenomenon, possibly involving poor nutrition, pollution, overexposure to certain foods and alcohol, overuse of antibiotics, stress and food additives. Removing identified trigger foods might help the immune system to recover, but other factors also need to be dealt with to heal the gut in order to have a major impact on long-term food intolerance.

Food addiction

One interesting finding among people with food intolerances is that they often become hooked on the very food that causes a reaction. This can lead to bingeing on the foods that harm them the most. Many patients describe these foods as leaving them feeling drugged or dopey. In some cases the foods induce a mild state of euphoria. In this way, the food can act as a psychological escape mechanism from uncomfortable situations. But why do some foods cause drug-like reactions?

When pain no longer serves a purpose as part of a survival mechanism, chemicals called endorphins are released. These are the body's natural painkillers – they make you feel good. The way they do this is by binding to sites that turn off pain and turning on pleasant sensations. Opiates, such as morphine, are similar in chemical structure and bind to the same sites, which is why they suppress pain.

These endorphins, whether made by the body or taken as a drug, are peptides. Peptides are small groups of amino acids bound together – smaller than a protein and larger than an amino acid. When the protein that you eat is digested, it first becomes peptides and then, if digestion works well, single amino acids. In the laboratory, endorphin-like peptides have been made from wheat, milk, barley and corn using human digestive enzymes. These peptides have been shown to bind to endorphin receptor sites triggering a 'feel-good' effect.

In addition, if foods to which you are intolerant are eaten, there is evidence that special cells in the gut release more serotonin (our happy hormone) to make the gut move faster – in other words, to cause diarrhoea, so that the gut is emptied of the noxious food. If serotonin is released in the blood faster than it can be absorbed, the level of free serotonin in the blood will be increased and that will make you feel good.

Preliminary research does seem to show that certain foods, most commonly wheat and milk, might induce a short-term positive feeling, even if, in the long term, they are causing health problems. Too often, the foods that don't suit you are the ones that you feel you 'couldn't live without'. This is exactly what happens in the case of many food intolerances. If you stop eating the suspect food, you might feel worse for a few days before you feel better. Some foods are addictive in their own right, such as sugar, alcohol, coffee, chocolate and tea (especially Earl Grey, which contains bergamot). You can react to these foods without being allergic or intolerant. Wheat, corn and milk could be added to this list on the basis of their endorphin-like effects.

How can you reverse a food intolerance?

Whatever the contributing causes, the first step is to identify the foods that are causing a problem (don't try to guess), and then avoid those foods you react strongly to. You can 'rotate' those foods that produce a mild reaction, which means that you eat them not more than once in every five days. (If you eat a reactive food every day, your level of reactivity will build up.) (See Resources for more about getting help to do this correctly.)

The good news is that IgG antibody reactions often go away if you: (a) avoid the food strictly for three to four months; and (b) heal the gut. This is because the cells that produce IgG antibodies have a half-life of six weeks, so six weeks later there will be half as many. The 'memory' of these antibodies is short term, and within six months there is not likely to be any residual memory of reaction to a food that's been avoided. Although a six-month avoidance period might be ideal, allergy expert Dr James Braly reports good results after as little as a month. Another option, after strict one-month avoidance, is to rotate foods as explained above so that an IgG-sensitive food is eaten only once every four days. This reduces the build-up of allergen-antibody complexes and reduces the chances of symptoms of intolerance. Foods such as wheat and milk, which commonly cause intolerances, are not a necessary part of our diet and can be avoided permanently without any health problems. It is important not to remove foods just for the sake of it, however, because you can limit your diet and therefore risk reducing the nutrients you need to be healthy; for example, if you do eliminate dairy products, as I do, you'll need to eat nuts and seeds, and plenty of vegetables to get enough calcium.

The same is not true for IgE classic allergic reactions, however. With regard to foods that provoke an IgE-type, immediate and pronounced reaction, these will probably need to be avoided for life because the memory of IgE antibodies is long term. As mentioned earlier, I have an IgE allergy to milk. I always react to it even if I haven't had any for a year, and even though there are things I can do to reduce the severity of the reaction – for example, by supplementing anti-inflammatory nutrients such as quercetin, glutamine, vitamin C, MSM (sulphur) and bromelain (the enzyme in pineapple).

We often develop food intolerances because the gut wall becomes inflamed or damaged, allowing incompletely digested food proteins to enter the bloodstream. The gut wall is also damaged by alcohol, painkillers, or too much coffee and fried foods.

Certain foods irritate the gut wall. An example is wheat, which contains gliadin, as explained in Chapter 9. This is why a lot of people are somewhat intolerant of wheat. Ancient wheat, in contrast, contains different kinds of gliadin, which might not be so reactive.

Fortunately, the cells that line the gut wall heal and replenish very quickly, especially when you feed them an amino acid called L-glutamine, so supplementing L-glutamine can speed up gut healing. If you want to heal a leaky gut, take 5g (a heaped teaspoon) of glutamine powder in cold water (not hot, because heat destroys this amino acid) last thing at night or at least half an hour before eating.

Summary – Chapter 10

If you have a food intolerance, try the following:

- Take digestive enzymes with each meal.
- Take probiotics daily for at least two weeks.
- Identify and avoid your food intolerances. Reintroduce offending foods one by one after three months, eating them infrequently, ideally no more than every four days, to minimise the chance of becoming intolerant to the food once more.
- Take a teaspoon of glutamine (5g) daily, away from food, for at least two weeks.

CHAPTER 11

Do You Have the Guts to be Happy and Stress-Free?

When you feel tired, depressed, stressed or anxious, it's unlikely that you would think that your digestive system, or something you've eaten, could be connected to it in any way. Yet most strong feelings are physically felt somewhere along the digestive tract. We feel emotions in our gut and often experience them affecting our appetite and our ability to digest properly. It's all part of a normal evolutionary reaction. When you're sick, injured, stressed or down, you want to effectively retreat into your 'cave' to recover your strength to face the world. That recovery has a lot more to do with what happens in your gut than you might think.

Your second brain

Today, science is discovering stronger connections between the brain and body than were earlier understood. The digestive system seems to act like a second brain, producing neurotransmitters, hormones and immune-transmitters, called cytokines, that cross-communicate with the brain. These cytokines have receptors on both the immune cells and the brain cells. We now know that every emotion we experience has a direct biological effect, activating the nervous, endocrine and immune systems.

The same is true with every piece of food you eat. The gut lining, which makes up a surface area about the size of a tennis court and half the thickness of a sheet of paper, is the interface between you and your food, and it is programmed to react against anything eaten just in case it is a foe. Ninety-nine per cent of the time, however, a healthy immune system – which is more active in the gut than anywhere else – switches off that reaction.

Eating certain foods can help that 'switching-off' mechanism. These are the omega-3 fats from fish and seeds such as chia, flax and pumpkin.[77] They stop the gut becoming inflamed and they also halt psychological inflammation, which causes feelings of aggression, irritability and depression – a condition that is sometimes anger turned inward.

It might surprise you to learn that any gut-related problem has a direct effect on your brain. But when you think of the gut as the interface between the exterior world and your body – and our experience of life as the interaction between the exterior world, perceived through our senses, and how we interpret them – it makes sense that your gut and your brain effectively 'talk' to each other.

The vagal nerve is a super-neural highway that connects the brain and gut directly. When you have inflammation – either in the gut or elsewhere in the body – the cytokines, activated by gut reactions, communicate with your brain to put you into 'retreat' mode and, in effect, make you want to hide away until you feel better. Likewise, stress has a direct effect on your gut, making your digestive system less tolerant.

Cytokines can make you feel depressed, and they have direct effects on the mood-boosting neurotransmitter serotonin. In fact, the vast majority of serotonin made in the body is made in a healthy gut.

The role of gut bacteria

An imbalance or depletion of bacteria in the gut has a similar effect to that of cytokines and might also influence our mood. As we saw in Chapter 7, we have considerably more bacteria in the gut than we have cells in our entire body, and they are absolutely vital for proper immunity. Probiotics (supplements of good bacteria) help to promote and 'train' cytokines to do their job properly. In so doing, they not only calm down inflammation in the gut, but they also help to signal to the brain to calm down, reducing stress reactions. Probiotics also boost something called 'brain-derived neurotrophic factor', which makes the brain's receptors more responsive to neurotransmitters. Research has found that supplementing probiotics has been shown to improve mood in those who are prone to depression.[78]

Brain allergies

As we saw in Chapter 9, a wheat intolerance can be the cause of schizophrenia symptoms, but most people wouldn't think of food allergies as a potential cause of this or, more ordinarily, of tiredness, low mood, poor concentration and anxiety. Yet the knowledge that an allergy to foods and chemicals can adversely affect moods and behaviour in susceptible individuals has been known for a very long time. Food allergies have been proven to cause a diverse range of symptoms including chronic fatigue, slowed thought processes, lack of motivation, irritability, agitation, aggressive behaviour, nervousness, anxiety, depression, alcoholism and substance abuse, schizophrenia, hyperactivity (ADHD), panic attacks, autism and various learning disabilities.[79]

A doctor from Munich, Joseph Egger, was one of the first pioneers to study the link between allergy and mental health. He decided to test 30 patients suffering from anxiety, depression, confusion or difficulty in concentrating for allergies, using a double-blind placebo-controlled trial. He gave the patients either dummy foods or foods that were allergenic to them, in small quantities, disguised so that they didn't know what they were eating. The results showed that the food allergens alone were able to produce severe depression, nervousness, feelings of anger without a particular object, loss of motivation and severe mental blankness. The foods that produced the most severe mental reactions were wheat, milk, cane sugar and eggs.[80]

Another pioneer of food and chemical sensitivity was Dr Benjamin Feingold, whose Feingold Diet became famous in the 1970s. He investigated the possibility of food allergies and sensitivity to salicylates (a compound used in aspirin) in 96 patients diagnosed as suffering from alcohol dependence, major depressive disorders and schizophrenia compared to 62 control subjects selected from adult hospital staff members for a possible food or chemical intolerance. The results showed that the group of patients diagnosed as depressives had the highest number of allergies: 80 per cent were allergic to grains, and all were allergic to egg white. Only 9 per cent of the control group were found to suffer from any allergies.[81]

As we saw in Chapter 9, many people are gluten intolerant. An exceedingly common symptom of celiac sufferers, the most severe kind of gluten intolerance, is depression.[82] Also, you don't have to have celiac disease or gut damage to react to wheat gluten. It can simply cause neurological problems such as depression, headache or migraine.[83]

These studies are prime examples of how problems created by food allergies or intolerances can produce a multitude of mental as well as physical symptoms, because they affect the central nervous system, and even the whole body. The state of inflammation, potentially induced by an allergic reaction, is found in many mental-health conditions, including depression[84] and is probably one of the main mechanisms by which a food allergy affects the brain. What is more, allergies are very specific to the individual, as are the symptoms they create, so any diagnosis can only be made individually by proper food-allergy testing.

The Brain Bio Centre is an outpatient clinic of the charitable Food for the Brain Foundation, which I set up ten years ago to treat people with mental-health issues using nutritional therapy. At the Centre we routinely test individuals for allergies and intolerances who are experiencing low mood or low motivation. It is not at all uncommon for us to find that putting a person on the allergy-free diet they need relieves symptoms of depression, insomnia or anxiety. If you suffer from poor concentration, insomnia, anxiety or other symptoms of depleted mental health, it's well worth investigating whether food allergies or intolerances play a part.

Case Study: Philip

When Philip came to the Brain Bio Centre he had had a long history of mental-health problems and years of trying various antidepressants. He had experienced severe periods of depression and sometimes had suicidal thoughts, along with many unpleasant side effects from the medication he was taking. He felt he wanted to be able to 'enjoy life to the full' but wasn't able to.

When we tested him for IgG-based food intolerances, he reacted to many foods, including gluten, egg white, corn and barley. After removing these foods from his diet, and by introducing a supplement programme to support his general health, he began to experience fewer spells of feeling down and had noticed what he described as a 'huge improvement' in his general well-being and mood.

Philip did experience a bad patch, while he was on holiday. He had strayed from his usually healthy diet and eaten a lot of the foods he was intolerant to, and his symptoms started to return. But as soon as he got his diet back on track he almost immediately began to feel better again. He has now started working and feels as though he has accomplished his goal of enjoying life.

Why stress shuts down digestion

Three in four people in Britain frequently feel stressed, with declining energy levels, and two in three experience frequent anxiety and tension, according to a UK survey of 51,000 people.[85] Chronic stress has dire long-term health consequences, increasing the risk of heart disease by five times[86] and doubling the risk of obesity, dementia and diabetes.[87] In fact, chronic stress is as bad for you as smoking, according to a study in the *Journal of the American Medical Association*.[88] Twenty-first-century living puts us on high alert. The average person checks their mobile phone every ten minutes and answers work-related emails on holiday. One in ten young adults even admits to checking their mobile phone during sex! Being constantly on the go is draining, with one in five Brits now needing to take time off work due to the ill effects of stress.[89]

The very same 'fight, flight, freeze' mechanism designed to promote our ancestors' survival – while they were hunting and being hunted by predators – shuts down digestion. After all, when your life is on the line, which is what the adrenal glands (which make and release stress hormones) assume, why waste energy digesting food? Immunity is also shut down, with all available energy being diverted into better muscle function, sharper vision, deeper breathing and liberating stores of glucose for energy.

Although modern stresses are rarely life threatening, they are far more frequent and relentless. Feeling overwhelmed at work, with money or relationship worries, being stuck in traffic, for example, can all cause the body to release the stress hormones adrenalin and cortisol, and to keep releasing them hour after hour.

When you go into a state of stress, hormones feed your state back to the gut, shutting down digestion and promoting inflammation. This happens, for example, when baby rats are separated from their mother.[90] However, research has found that giving probiotics reduces this stress response and helps reset the system out of stress.[91] Taking probiotics helps to reduce levels of adrenal hormones and, by reducing inflammation, switch your body away from a reactive state. Digestive enzymes also help to do this.

Prolonged stress, marked by high levels of cortisol and

low levels of the hormone DHEA (dihydroepiandrosterone), depresses immunity. Think of it as the bouncers going on strike at a nightclub. The bouncers in this case are called secretory IgA (or SIgA, secretory immunoglobulin A); they line the digestive tract and their job is to protect the body from the entry of undesirable molecules. We lose this protection as SIgA levels fall when we are under stress, which results in large, undesirable molecules finding their way into the body. These stimulate an immune response – an allergic reaction – and this is why people under chronic stress are more likely to develop food sensitivities. (SIgA levels are often measured alongside cortisol and DHEA as part of an adrenal stress test.) Too much stress both suppresses the immune system and encourages inflammation, setting the scene for gastrointestinal infections and distress.

That's why it's harder to digest food when you're feeling stressed and why you become more prone to illnesses and find them harder to shift if that stress is prolonged. It's a vicious cycle because, if you don't eat well and digest your food efficiently, you won't get the nutrients to give you the energy to respond to the issues that trigger a stress reaction in the first place.

Don't drink coffee with food

A classic mistake that many people make is to combine an adrenal stimulant with food – starting the day, for example, with a coffee or strong tea (which are stimulants) and a croissant. Nicotine is also a stimulant and has a direct effect on the digestion by shutting it down. If you *have* to drink coffee (or smoke), do so away from food; for example, have a coffee in the morning, at least one hour before eating. Both smoking and coffee drinking as ways of giving you a boost become increasingly less necessary or desirable once you adopt a healthy, optimal diet and lifestyle and your natural energy levels increase.

Don't eat on the move

In our 24/7 society it is all too easy to cram work (and stress) into every minute, never taking time to slow down, chill out or enjoy your meals either on your own or with friends and family. This is in contrast to the Mediterranean style of eating, which involves taking time off to enjoy lunch. It is a much healthier way of existence.

As we learnt in Chapter 1, it is important to chew your food, thus taking more time to digest and absorb the nutrients within. A simple act of saying grace, or internally expressing your gratitude for the food on the table, is also a great way to remind yourself to slow down when eating. It is no coincidence that the very first line in the Lord's Prayer is: 'Give us this day our daily bread.'

In my book *The Stress Cure*, co-authored with Susannah Lawson, we talk about HeartMath, a simple practice of developing a stress-free way of being that involves a two-minute exercise called the Quick Coherence Technique. The HeartMath Institute has done some amazing research showing how to de-stress and build stress resilience, and also showing how damaging living in a state of constant stress is to many aspects of health, due to the high levels of adrenalin and cortisol it produces. This would be a very good exercise to do before eating, especially if you are caught in the stress trap. (See Resources for details, including a film that you can watch about the technique.)

Summary – Chapter 11

Next time you're feeling stressed or low, think about your digestive system:

- Take time to stop and eat in a relaxed fashion, perhaps practising the Quick Coherence Technique before eating, and express, internally, gratitude for the food on your plate.
- Don't drink coffee or strong tea with your meal.
- Might you be intolerant to a food? If you know to what, avoid it. Otherwise it might be worth getting yourself tested.
- Are you lacking in omega-3s from oily fish, chia, flax and pumpkin seeds?
- Have you been drinking alcohol, or taking painkillers or antibiotics?
- Might you benefit from taking some probiotics, glutamine or digestive enzymes to support your gut health? These are available in combination in some supplements and are worth taking for a month to help restore gut health (see Chapter 31).

PART III

DIGESTIVE PROBLEMS AND SOLUTIONS

CHAPTER 12

The Six Steps to Digestive Health

U nderlying most digestive disorders is disruption of the fundamental essentials of a healthy gut: a good diet to start with, backed up by good digestion and absorption, a diverse and healthy gut microbiota, good gut-wall integrity, an absence of gut inflammation and food intolerances, and good elimination.

If you have started to follow the suggestions in Parts I and II of this book, your digestion is probably already much improved and your digestive symptoms will have been reduced. This is because most digestive problems are a consequence of one or more of the following issues:

- Poor digestion (irritation, intoxication, lack of enzymes, lack of stomach acid).
- Poor absorption (increased gut permeability).
- Poor protection (dysbiosis, inflammation, food intolerances).
- Poor elimination (clogged up colon, liver-detoxification problems).

This common sequence of events is shown below, together with the remedial actions necessary to get everything working properly again. These form the basis of my programme to restore digestive health, explained in more detail in Part IV.

What goes wrong and how to correct it

Do you have...

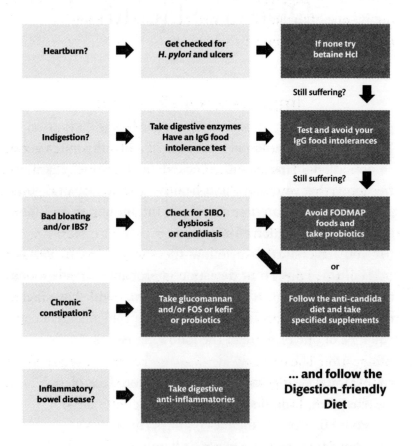

The following chapters explore the most common digestive problems that affect almost everyone at some time in their lives, giving exact strategies for their resolution.

One survey found that almost 70 per cent of US households experience a digestive disorder.[1] To a very real extent, digestive problems are a silent epidemic and a major cause of discomfort in our modern world. The consequences of having digestive problems are much more far-reaching than most of us realise and they can lead to arthritis, chronic fatigue, headaches and migraines, sinus problems, eczema, psoriasis, infections and many other common diseases not usually connected to digestion. Restoring digestive health is, without doubt, one of the keys to a long, healthy and happy life. Here's a crash course in how to achieve it.

Improve your digestion

Step 1 is to eat the right foods, in the correct amounts and combinations. This means eating whole, unrefined, chemical-free foods that your digestive system is designed to work with, digest and absorb. What this means exactly is explained in Part IV, and you will find recipes that meet with these criteria in Part V. By now, however, I suspect you're getting the gist of the kind of diet I'll be recommending: one that is free from modern wheat and the digestive irritants that I described in the previous section of the book.

Indigestion The easiest way to test and correct indigestion is simply to take a digestive enzyme supplement with each meal for one week. Find one that provides the following:

- Amylase – to digest carbs
- Invertase – to digest sugars
- Protease – to digest protein
- Lipase – to digest fats

- Alpha-galactosidase – to digest pulses
- Glucoamylase (also called amylo-glucosidase) – to digest greens
- Lactase – to digest dairy products

If you find substantial relief, keep going for as long as you need to, or adjust as necessary to take with your main meals only or when you eat foods you find hard to digest, such as beans or greens.

If you are still experiencing indigestion or heartburn, read Chapter 17 on stopping GERD and acid reflux, as well as Chapter 4 on passing the acid test.

Improve your absorption

Step 2 is to improve your gut integrity. The easiest and fastest way to do this is by taking two teaspoons of L-glutamine powder, one teaspoon at night, in water, just before you go to bed, and one teaspoon on rising, waiting an hour before you eat. Do this for one week.

If you have been diagnosed with leaky gut syndrome, read Chapter 15 on reversing the condition.

Improve your protection

Step 3 is to re-inoculate your gut with healthy bacteria. The cornerstones of good gut microbiota are *Lactobacillus* and *Bifidobacterium*. For one week, supplement 2–5 billion viable organisms a day, ideally twice a day. Also, avoid alcohol. Read Chapter 7 to find out more about these probiotic bacteria.

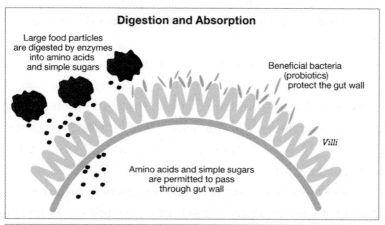

Digestion and Absorption

Large food particles are digested by enzymes into amino acids and simple sugars

Beneficial bacteria (probiotics) protect the gut wall

Villi

Amino acids and simple sugars are permitted to pass through gut wall

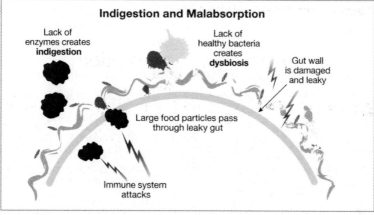

Indigestion and Malabsorption

Lack of enzymes creates **indigestion**

Lack of healthy bacteria creates **dysbiosis**

Gut wall is damaged and leaky

Large food particles pass through leaky gut

Immune system attacks

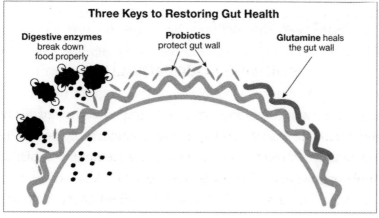

Three Keys to Restoring Gut Health

Digestive enzymes break down food properly

Probiotics protect gut wall

Glutamine heals the gut wall

Three steps to digestive health

Calm inflammation down

Step 4 If your gut is in an inflamed state, the best way to calm it down is to eat a healthy diet, free from foods that you are intolerant to. The following can help to calm down a belligerent hyperactive GALT (gut associated lymphatic system):

Omega-3 fish oils Eat oily fish two or three times a week and supplement at least 1,000mg of omega-3 fish oil daily providing at least 333mg (a third) EPA, which is the most anti-inflammatory omega-3. Also eat chia seeds – this is especially important for vegans.

Turmeric Of all the natural painkillers and anti-inflammatories, turmeric is the best all-rounder. Although it can act locally in the gut, it is, however, poorly absorbed. Various new forms of turmeric, concentrating the active ingredient, curcumin, and delivering this in an absorbable form, have improved its function by over one hundredfold. My favourite to switch off inflammation is turmeric oil, taken with each meal.

Quercetin with bromelain Quercetin is a potent anti-inflammatory found especially in red onions but also other foods. A red onion provides almost 20mg, but I like to take between 500mg and 1,000mg, equivalent to 50 red onions, to calm down gut inflammation. I aim to eat a red onion every day. Quercetin's absorption is considerably helped by bromelain, the protein-digesting enzyme in pineapple, so combinations of these two work best.

MSM (sulphur) Sulphur, found in onions, garlic and eggs, is vital for healthy methylation, which is a 'master control' function of the body, also required for nutrient absorption. It helps to heal a leaky gut and calms down inflammation. MSM is the most usable form of sulphur, readily absorbed, but also immediately helping to calm down an inflamed gut.

Vitamin C is a natural anti-histamine. Histamine is released when the body reacts in an inflammatory way, so vitamin C helps to calm this down. People with incredibly sensitive digestive systems may need to take an alkaline form of this slightly acid vitamin, such as magnesium ascorbate. Magnesium also works as an anti-spasmodic.

You can buy combined supplements of the last three, but both omega-3 fish oils and turmeric oil cannot be combined in one pill, so you'll need to take these separately for one week initially to calm down inflammation. Read more about this in Chapter 16 'Fire Belly – Resolving Gut Inflammation'.

Eliminate food intolerances

Step 5 As we saw in Chapter 10, your body might have developed sensitivities and intolerances to certain foods that currently trigger an immune-based antibody response. When under attack, often the first step is to surrender, to calm down the situation. Get yourself tested for IgG antibody reactions against foods, then, in the short term, eliminate them. Chapter 10 explains when and how you can gradually reintroduce them, and then re-test your intolerances, which will decrease as you become healthier.

Improve elimination

Step 6 Finally, to encourage healthy elimination, increase your intake of soluble fibres, as explained in Chapter 6. You can do this using diet alone; for example, by eating more oat-based foods and chia seeds. However, if elimination is a sticking point for you, you might want to take a teaspoon (5g), or the equivalent number of capsules, of glucomannan or a glucomannan-based soluble fibre, always with a large glass of water immediately before each meal. This is also a good way to remind yourself to drink plenty of water – the equivalent of six glasses of water a day, including your hot drinks, is my recommendation. Vitamin C also helps to move things along. I recommend taking 2g of vitamin C a day.

If you're still 'stuck', read Chapter 27 about how to solve constipation, diverticulitis and haemorrhoids.

Before I give you the natural alternatives to solving various common digestive issues, in the next chapter I'd like to put their effectiveness into context by looking at the pros and cons – mainly cons – of the common drugs prescribed for various digestive disorders. Most of these will become unnecessary once you tune up your gut health by following the advice in this book.

Summary – Chapter 12

To restore good digestive health, you are going to need to address the six fundamental steps explained above:

- Eat a healthy diet.
- Ensure good digestion by taking digestive enzymes.
- Ensure good gut integrity by taking glutamine powder.
- Re-inoculate your gut by taking probiotics.
- Reduce inflammation with omega-3 fats and anti-inflammatory nutrients (turmeric, MSM, quercetin and vitamin C).
- Eliminate your food intolerances.
- Increase your intake of soluble fibres, primarily from oats and chia.

CHAPTER 13

The Truth about Digestion Drugs

H ippocrates is considered the father of modern medicine because he asked the simple question about diseases: what's the cause? Today, doctors no longer have to swear the Hippocratic Oath, which includes the maxim 'first do no harm'. Coincidentally, too many conventional approaches to digestive problems ignore the cause and just target relieving the symptoms. It is extraordinary how often I've heard people say that their doctors told them diet had nothing to do with their digestive disorder! Before we explore nutritional solutions to digestive problems it's worth understanding the pros and cons of the most often-prescribed drugs for digestive problems and why relying on these is often not a viable solution, even if it gets you out of an immediate fix. At the top of the list are antacids.

Antacids

Many people are diagnosed with GERD (gastro-oesophageal reflux disease), the main symptom of which is heartburn. Heartburn occurs when acid creeps out of the stomach and up into the oesophagus, the tube leading to the mouth, causing anything from a mild burning sensation to extreme discomfort. An estimated 40 per cent of Americans suffer from it at any one time. Pills that reduce the acid are an easy and effective solution. The most frequently used are a class of drugs called proton pump inhibitors (PPIs). PPIs are also given for gastrointestinal damage in people who regularly take aspirin-like NSAIDs (non-steroidal anti-inflammatory drugs). Given the number of people suffering from these conditions, it adds up to a good recipe for a blockbuster drug. However, even if you are familiar with claims against drug companies, what happened with two of the PPIs still comes as a shock. One of them, Propulsid (also known as cisapride), was sold for years despite information about its dangers being known, while the other, Nexium, was launched as a new drug costing ten times as much as the one it replaced, even though it was virtually chemically identical.

What happened with Propulsid is described in detail in a major investigation by the *New York Times*, published on 10 June 2005. The drug was granted a licence for heartburn in 1993 but by 1995, the FDA had evidence that it was linked to cases of severe disruption to heart rhythm. By 1998, the Propulsid-linked death toll was numbered in the dozens, and about a hundred people were believed to have suffered serious heart problems. However, the drug continued to be promoted until it was finally withdrawn in 2000, following the threat of a public hearing. At that point, the toll was estimated at 80 heart-related deaths and 341 injuries.[2]

In 2004, the parent company, Johnson & Johnson, agreed to settle outstanding claims at a total cost of $90 million. Many of the details in the *New York Times* piece came from documents the company had been required to release by the courts. No other PPI is currently said to pose this sort of risk – but if it did, how would we know?

It is also hard to see where science or benefit to patients comes into the launch of Nexium in 2003. Nexium replaced another PPI, Prilosec, as its patent was just about to run out; however, Nexium was chemically very similar to Prilosec, so it was hard to show that it was worth paying ten times the price for. Three studies compared the two, but two found no difference and one found that 90 per cent of the ulcers in patients on Nexium had healed after eight weeks, compared with 87 per cent for those on Prilosec. This was despite the fact that in these studies, the participants were getting double the dose of Nexium. However, a $257 million advertising campaign ensured that Nexium was widely prescribed, and sales are now running at $4.4 billion (2014 data).

A frequently wrongly prescribed drug

As you'll see in Chapter 17, these PPI drugs are often wrongly prescribed to people who are underproducing stomach acid, which leads to belching and acid reflux. These drugs are also widely used for stomach ulcers, indigestion and heartburn. Ironically, they are also given as the medical solution to the gut damage caused by long-term use of NSAID painkillers. PPIs are widely prescribed to prevent gastric bleeding in hospital patients, despite studies showing that over 700 people have to be treated for one person to benefit.[3] The NHS spends about half a billion pounds on them annually. Unfortunately, much of that is a waste of money because these drugs are heavily overprescribed. In fact, between 25 per cent and 70 per cent of those prescriptions have no medical basis.[4] This isn't just a waste, it also exposes patients to the inevitable serious side effects, which include pneumonia, osteoporosis, kidney disease and an increased risk of Alzheimer's.[5]

PPI drugs, and others like them, such as the histamine antagonists called H2RAs, suppress stomach secretion, which inhibits vitamin B_{12} absorption, thereby increasing a risk of deficiency. Vitamin B_{12} cannot be absorbed without combining with 'intrinsic factor' excreted by the stomach. More than 1.5 PPI pills per day doubles the risk of B_{12} deficiency, concluded a study in the *Journal of the American Medical Association*.[6] Our body's ability to absorb vitamins declines as we get older, but vitamin B_{12} absorption decreases more rapidly than the others. One in five older people have insufficient blood levels of B_{12} to prevent premature brain shrinkage.[7] Why this happens isn't fully understood, although certainly a lack of stomach acid (known as achlorhydria) is one reason, although indigestion and heartburn can also be caused by having too much stomach acid. Low production might be linked to a lack of zinc, as we saw in Chapter 4, which is needed to make stomach acid. Many people get acid reflux, which is essentially a mechanical problem, even though they underproduce stomach acid.

B_{12} deficiency, in turn, increases the risk of Alzheimer's, dementia and bone-mass loss. These drugs are also known to increase the risk of fracture, doubling the risk in those over 50 if taken in the long term, according to a study in the *Journal of the American Medical Association*.[8] The usual reason given is because lower acid interferes with calcium absorption, as well as other vital minerals such as magnesium. But the negative effect that they have on B_{12} – which is needed for methylation, which in turn is needed to build bones – might be adding to the problem. Anyone considering taking, or anyone who is already taking, these drugs should have their homocysteine and B_{12} levels checked regularly. (Homocysteine is a marker in the blood that rises if the body doesn't have enough B vitamins, such as B_{12}. This might be a consequence of poor absorption rather than lack of these vitamins in the diet.)

PPIs might also increase your risk of being infected by the superbug *Clostridium difficile* if you go into hospital, because a normal amount of stomach acid kills off the bacterium.[9] PPIs also increase the risk of developing pneumonia by 1½ times.[10] With less stomach acid, the odds of developing dysbiosis increase.

Apart from the risks linked to PPIs, which are usually prescribed for the symptoms of making too much acid, as we have seen, many people diagnosed with GERD and heartburn actually *lack* stomach acid and benefit from supplementing it. See Chapter 17 to find out how to stop GERD and acid reflux.

Painkillers and anti-inflammatories

Almost everyone takes an aspirin or some other NSAID (non-steroidal anti-inflammatory drug), such as ibuprofen, occasionally with little chance of harm. Indeed, the average person takes 373 painkillers a year, according to one survey.[11] However, used regularly, for chronic conditions such as arthritis and joint pain, these drugs are famously linked with an increased risk of bleeding and damage to the small intestine.[12] American figures estimate this causes 103,000 hospitalisations and 16,500 deaths a year.[13] In the UK several thousand deaths from intestinal bleeding caused by NSAIDs are recorded every year. Even so, NSAIDs are widely used in the long term – 70 per cent of people over the age of 65 take them at least once a week, and nearly half of those take seven doses or more per week.[14] This is in spite of the fact that, for reducing arthritic knee pain for longer than a few weeks, NSAIDs are little better than a placebo.[15]

If you are in pain, it is understandable that you would want to take a painkiller, but your body is trying to tell you something, and it is vital to explore the underlying cause of the pain rather than simply suppressing the actual pain. Codeine-based painkillers tell your brain to suppress pain, and frequent use can lead to dependence. Paracetamol/acetaminophen works but is hard work on the liver, as I explain in Chapter 25. NSAIDs do reduce inflammation, but they also damage the gut – some types more than others. (See Chapter 16 for how to reverse gut inflammation.)

New drugs, same problems?

Because many of these drugs are off-patent – which means that the pharmaceutical companies that first developed them no longer have the sole right to sell them and they can now be sold cheaply as generic brands – so there's no more big money to be made from them. Consequently, there's a whole new class of anti-inflammatory drugs prescribed for inflammatory bowel diseases, including Crohn's and ulcerative colitis, the top two being Humira (adalimumab) worth $1.56 billion per quarter and Remicade (infliximab), which, combined, accounted for $23 billion in global sales in 2014.

The list of side effects for Humira and Remicade is too long to include, but you can see it yourself by going to www.rxlist.com, selecting the drug, then going to its 'side effects centre'. A very useful and impartial website for patients and doctors to report their reactions is www.rxisk.org. It's a good place to check out any dangers with drugs you might be prescribed. The website is run by Dr David Healy, who blew the whistle on antidepressants causing suicidal tendencies. He is also author of *Pharmageddon*. Dr Healy's blog explores the use of Humira in ulcerative colitis, and people can use it to report their experiences with the drug.[16]

A new drug called vedolizumab is soon to be launched. Its results are said to be as good as Humira's, but with far fewer side effects. Only time will tell, as the same claim has been made for many new medications that were introduced once the patent of a former one ran out.

In suppressing immune-system reactions these drugs can pave the way for sometimes life-threatening infections and cancers. Before you take them, my advice is to try everything in this book first. The important question to address is: why is my immune system overreacting? Simply suppressing it ignores this question, which is key to solving any autoimmune disease.

Antibiotics

The sacred cow of modern medicine, antibiotics were the first blockbuster drugs that saved, and continue to save, millions of lives. Their discovery gave birth to the idea that there would be a miracle drug for each disease and spawned the now trillion-dollar pharmaceutical industry.

There is a problem, however. The widespread overuse of antibiotics, both for humans and in animal feed, has paved the way for the emergence of superbugs that are resistant to antibiotics, and these claim an increasing number of lives each year. Geoffrey Cannon first wrote convincingly about this in his book *Superbugs: Nature's Revenge*, which predicted exactly what is happening now.

There is not as much of a financial incentive for pharmaceutical companies in developing new antibiotics, because they are taken by patients for only a short while, not on a daily basis over many years, which is obviously much more profitable. As a result, there are insufficient new antibiotics available to counteract new and stronger strains of bacteria.

Fighting infection while nurturing your gut

If you succumb to a gut infection, try to avoid using anti-biotics and follow the recommendations in Chapter 21, but if you do need to take them be aware of the downsides too and be prepared to act to alleviate them.

Antibiotics wipe out the beneficial bacteria in the gut at the same time that they kill the pathogenic bacteria, leading to a growth in undesirable bacteria and increasing intestinal permeability.[17] Further infection is thus more likely, as is increased gut inflammation. In animal studies, the largest changes in the gut microbiota have been found from using amoxicillin and vancomycin, popular broad-spectrum anti-biotics, and the least from using metronidazole, which is effective against a number of gut infections (see Chapter 21). Some stronger antibiotics, such as fluoroquinolones, are asso-ciated with horrendous side effects. The UK's drug watchdog, the Medicines and Healthcare Products Regulatory Authority (MHRA), says that 5,962 adverse drug reactions have been reported in the UK since 1990 for fluoroquinolones, with more than 4,500 for ciprofloxacin, the most frequently pre-scribed fluoroquinolone (although these might be seriously underreported).[18]

Your doctor will advise you which antibiotic is the most effective against your kind of infection. It is certainly a ter-rible idea to take long-term antibiotics for conditions such as acne, which are resolvable with an optimum-nutrition approach.

It is therefore essential to take probiotic supplements both during antibiotic treatment and for two to four weeks afterwards to restore a healthy level and population of gut bacteria. Take the probiotics away from the antibiotics, twice a day. It is best to choose a combination of several strains of

Lactobacillus and bifidobacteria, consuming at least 10 billion viable organisms a day, so look for a supplement that gives at least 5 billion viable organisms per capsule.

If you or your doctor suspect you have small intestinal bacterial overgrowth (SIBO – see page 149), the best antibiotic to take is Rifaximin. Is it not absorbed through the gut wall, so it acts locally, killing off bad bacteria. It has proven to be effective in reducing symptoms of bacterial overgrowth[19] with rare adverse effects.[20]

Anti-spasmodics and laxatives

A traumatised digestive system loses its most basic function, which is to defecate after meals. Ideally, this should happen two or three times a day. Instead, most people are constipated, while others have the opposite problem, with too frequent and urgent defecation. (See how to solve these problems in Chapters 22, 26 and 27.)

Meanwhile, millions of prescriptions are written for laxatives and anti-spasmodics, with 15 per cent of the Western population classified as constipated, although the Holford 100% Health Survey of 2011 showed that nine out of ten people don't move their bowels every day.[21]

Anti-spasmodics are a group of medicines that help to control gut spasm. The two main types are anti-muscarinics, such as dicycloverine, hyoscine and atropine, and smooth-muscle relaxants such as alverine and mebeverine. There are natural anti-spasmodics, however, such as peppermint oil and berberine, an extract found in various herbs such as goldenseal. My favourite is peppermint oil.

Laxatives work in different ways. There are those that act as bulking agents based on highly absorbent fibres. Metamucil and Citrucel fall into this category. I prefer PGX or glucomannan, the super-soluble fibre, always taken with a large glass of water (see Chapter 6). These are less harmful, and are even beneficial for the digestive system. Also worth a mention are osmotics, such as Milk of Magnesia, which draw water into the colon from surrounding tissues, thus making it easier to move the material along.

More concerning are those laxatives that work by triggering rhythmic contractions of intestinal muscles to promote a bowel movement. These can be given orally, such as Dulcolax or Senokot, or as suppositories, such as Bisacodyl, Pedia-Lax and Dulcolax.

You *do* want rhythmic bowel contractions, but naturally, usually after meals – a bodily function that we have already looked at called peristalsis. (In Chapter 27 I talk about how to encourage your own natural peristalsis.) The problem with forcing these contractions, especially on a regular basis, is that your body can lose its own natural rhythm. A diet low in fibre, making it harder to move material along, a lack of water and vitamin C, and too much caffeine can all contribute to the loss of natural peristalsis.

Summary – Chapter 13

Stay off drugs for digestive disorders as much as you can, with the exception of antibiotics when needed for a serious gut infection, and first explore the specific strategies outlined in this book, depending on your condition. Drugs should be a last resort, when all nutritional avenues have been exhausted.

CHAPTER 14

Dealing with Dysbiosis

When the balance of healthy bacteria in the digestive tract is disrupted and unhealthy bacteria
take over, this is called 'dysbiosis'. The term
dysbiosis was coined at the beginning of the last century by
Dr Eli Metchnikoff, who succeeded Louis Pasteur as the director of the Pasteur Institute in Paris. He proposed that many
digestive diseases resulted from an imbalance of microorganisms in the digestive tract. Even though he won a Nobel Prize
in 1908 for his work on the beneficial role of lactobacilli in
boosting immunity, modern medicine essentially ignored his
work in favour of producing antibiotics and other microbe-
killing drugs. As a result, many disease-causing microbes
have become resistant to drugs, becoming superbugs, as we
saw in the previous chapter. Superbugs now exist for staphylococcus (MRSA) and streptococcus infections, gonorrhoea,
leprosy and tuberculosis, *Clostridium difficile* and enterococci,
and the list is growing. Many other bacteria have become
resistant to specific types of antibiotics, and tens of thousands
of people now die every year because no antibiotic can be
found to treat their drug-resistant infections.

Understanding dysbiosis isn't about defining a new disease.

Rather, it involves redefining the underlying cause of many diseases and reconsidering their method of treatment.

Virtually every disease discussed in this book has dysbiosis as an underlying root cause, and every chapter so far has introduced one factor after another which, if ignored, will set the scene for dysbiosis.

The pathway to dysbiosis

A lack of enzymes, too little stomach acid, vitamin and mineral deficiencies, eating food allergens and inflammatory foods, taking certain drugs, exposure to disease-causing microbes, a lack of fibre, unhealthy intestinal flora – all these are the building blocks of dysbiosis. The symptoms are far-reaching because, once the digestive tract is no longer working properly, detoxification problems and inflammation are likely to follow.

Ironically, perhaps the greatest single contributors to dysbiosis are the very drugs used to treat the symptoms of these problems: antibiotics, steroids and, especially, non-steroidal anti-inflammatory drugs.

Steroid drugs feed candida infections (see Chapter 24), whereas non-steroidal drugs are highly irritating to the digestive tract. Antibiotics, especially broad-spectrum antibiotics such as amoxicillin, wipe out not only the bad guys but also the good guys, removing our ability to keep further infections at bay.

The use of these drugs can generate the very conditions that lead to infection or inflammation, for which the conventional answer is more of the same drug. This might be good for business, but it's not good for your health. To reverse dysbiosis it is essential to look at the whole picture, the entire ecology of the digestive environment. According to Elizabeth Lipski, author of *Digestive Wellness*, there are four kinds of dysbiosis:

1 **Putrefaction dysbiosis** is a consequence of food not being properly digested and eliminated, resulting in putrefaction and the generation of toxic by-products. The net result is bloating, discomfort and indigestion. This is the most common type of dysbiosis and the inevitable consequence of eating a high-fat, high-meat, low-fibre diet. This leads to too much bad bacteria (bacteroides) and too little good (bifidobacteria). The bacteroides break down vitamin B_{12}, so the person starts to experience deficiency symptoms, such as fatigue, depression and weakness. The bad bacteria also convert bile into all kinds of toxins associated with promoting cancer.

2 **Fermentation dysbiosis** is when the imbalance of micro-organisms favours those that ferment carbohydrate. Such people feel worse after eating carbohydrate or sugar-rich foods, which include fruit, beer, wine and grain products (such as bread or cereals).

3 **Deficiency dysbiosis** occurs when a person is deficient in beneficial bacteria, perhaps as a result of a course of antibiotics. Until their intestinal flora has returned to good health, they will be prone to irritable bowel syndrome, allergies and infections.

4 **Sensitisation dysbiosis** occurs when the gut-associated immune system becomes highly sensitised to substances both in food and those produced by microbes. Effectively, such a person becomes multi-allergic, and their symptoms are often systemic (that is, not just in the gut). It is highly likely that many sufferers of autoimmune diseases, such as rheumatoid

arthritis, lupus and possibly eczema and psoriasis, might fall into this category.

The solution is to find out exactly what's happening in a person's digestive ecosystem and then to put it right. To this end, a clinical nutritionist is likely to recommend a 'comprehensive digestive stool analysis'. This can determine how well a person is digesting and absorbing, and which of these four types of dysbiosis is present; for example, a high level of beta-glucoronidase indicates putrefaction dysbiosis, whereas a high level of the yeast *Candida albicans* points to fermentation dysbiosis. An absence of sufficient lactobacilli or bifidus bacteria indicates a deficiency dysbiosis that might respond to supplementing those probiotic bacteria. Abnormal levels of immunoglobulin A (IgA) can indicate sensitisation dysbiosis and a greater risk of allergies. Such tests can also identify the presence of UFOs (unfriendly faecal organisms), which are the subject of Chapter 21.

I'd like to add a fifth 'dysbiosis', called SIBO:

SIBO dysbiosis Many people now suffer from an overgrowth of unhealthy bacteria in the gut, especially in the small intestine, as a consequence of something 'upstream' not working properly, be it a lack of digestive enzymes, insufficient stomach acid or just too much lousy food. This is called small intestine bacterial overgrowth (SIBO). These unhealthy bacteria take over the gut microbiota and survive by eating your food and producing gas and bloating. This is a very common cause of irritable bowel syndrome, discussed in more detail in Chapter 23. We can consider candidiasis, the overgrowth of *Candida albicans*, as one specific type of SIBO, the symptoms of which also include bloating, especially after eating carbohydrates such as fruit.

*

There are many contributory causes of these different kinds of dysbiosis that have already been discussed in the book: use of antibiotics, antacids, anti-inflammatories, too much alcohol, caffeine, stress, poor eating habits (especially too much sugar), gut infections and food poisoning. Whatever the cause, what's the cure?

Restoring healthy gut bacteria

The best cure depends on your particular imbalance of gut bacteria, and that first requires a test. From a sample of your faeces it is possible to culture and find which organisms, good and bad, are present in your gut, and therefore devise the most effective probiotic 're-inoculation'. The goal here is to encourage the good bacteria which will then crowd out the bad. While re-inoculating, it is wise to stop feeding the bad bacteria with its favourite food, which is sugar (although it appears that xylose, which is a sugar found in stone fruits such as cherries and plums, called xylitol when it is crystallised, does not feed these bacteria).

The specific strains of bacteria that will be right for you depend on your specific dysbiosis but, in many cases, it is best to take a combination of *Lactobacillus* and bifidobacteria species. The most commonly given are *Lactobacillus acidophilus* and *Bifidobacterium bifidum*. Think A (for acidophilus) and B (for bifidum). The bacteria in yoghurt 'eat' the milk sugar, lactose, to produce lactic acid, which is why natural yoghurt is quite bitter. Many probiotic drinks have destroyed this sugar-free benefit by including usually one specific strain of bacteria – one that they 'own' – in a milky sugary drink. These are, of course, bad news if you are dairy intolerant or trying to avoid sugar.

Some yoghurts purposely use a *Lactobacillus* and bifidobacteria combo and often use 'AB' or 'BA' in their name or label. Some are dairy-free. Most are sugar-free. These are a good way to restore a healthy microbiota.

The most effective, and probably most cost effective, route is to directly supplement, in capsules or powder, a combination of gut-friendly bacteria. This usually works out cheaper because you take one or two capsules a day; however, the manufacture and storage of bacteria is tricky. They are grown in vast vats, fed with a prebiotic food and, at the height of their growth, are freeze-dried and stored in a refrigerator. Often, at this stage, a prebiotic is included, such as FOS, such that, when the capsule hits your warm and moist stomach, this activates the bacteria to feed off the prebiotic and start growing again.

This is one area where I'd recommend buying a reputable brand (see Resources for reputable suppliers), and not skimping on quality, as some surveys have reported that some probiotic supplements don't actually contain what they say they do. Also, the amount of viable organisms makes a big difference. As a rough guideline I'd recommend 1–2 billion viable organisms a day for maintaining a healthy gut microbiota and 5–10 billion for correcting dysbiosis or treatment of a condition. In Chapter 7 I explained which specific strains have been used to treat which specific conditions, but I will give further guidance on specific conditions in the relevant chapters in this section.

Needless to say, it is vital to follow the same guidelines given in Chapter 7 to promote healthy gut bacteria. Once achieved, it is not necessary to keep taking probiotic supplements since they will be resident inside you, feeding off the healthy foods you will be eating.

Summary – Chapter 14

To alleviate dysbiosis:

- Eat a more plant-based diet with at least half of what's on your plate at main meals being steamed or raw vegetables.
- Eat fermented foods, such as yoghurt, cottage cheese, miso, shoyu, sauerkraut and sourdough bread made with Kamut (see Resources).
- Take a probiotic supplement containing beneficial strains of bacteria as well as FOS on a regular basis, but not necessarily every day.
- Limit alcohol and take a probiotic supplement after excessive alcohol intake.
- Take a higher-dose probiotic supplement during, and for two to four weeks after, a course of antibiotics.

CHAPTER 15

Reversing Leaky Gut Syndrome

F oods that are normally considered to be healthy can also become toxins in the body if they are not digested or absorbed properly. We are designed to digest our food into simple molecules that can readily pass through the digestive tract and into the bloodstream, as explained in Chapter 1. If, however, a person doesn't digest their food properly, or if the gut wall becomes leaky, incompletely digested foods can enter the blood. There they are likely to alert immune 'scout' cells which treat them as invaders, triggering an allergic reaction, as I explained earlier. The ensuing battle results in a complex of chemicals that are themselves toxic and need to be cleaned up.

The integrity of the gut wall is therefore critical to our health, and our bodies work hard to maintain its proper permeability in the face of considerable assault on a daily basis. It is now recognised by gastrointestinal experts that this permeability, while remarkable in its complexity, is vulnerable and subject to change, depending on the integrity of the gut wall and the substances it is exposed to. Increased permeability, far from enhancing the transport of nutrients, allows the entrance of toxins and improperly digested food particles, which can give rise to a number of health problems associated with 'leaky gut syndrome'.[22]

The symptoms and conditions associated with leaky gut syndrome are:

acne
AIDS/HIV infection
arthritis (osteo-/rheumatoid)
autism
celiac disease
childhood hyperactivity
chronic fatigue syndrome
chronic pancreatitis
cystic fibrosis
depression, mood swings
diarrhoea/constipation
eczema
fatigue
food/chemical sensitivities
inflammatory bowel disease (Crohn's, chronic
    hepatitis, ulcerative colitis)
irritable bowel syndrome
psoriasis, dermatitis
urticaria (hives)
viral, bacterial or yeast infection

The lining of the digestive tract is a remarkably complex 'skin' which performs countless functions: digesting foods, absorbing them, moving food along, providing immune protection, and so on. Its folds, lined with villi (see page 40), perform the seemingly contradictory task of acting as both a barrier to toxins and large food particles, and a one-way selective gateway to nutrients. This careful balance is challenged every day by a host of toxins and allergens, which – with optimum health of the mucous membranes, proper permeability, immunity, liver function and flora – pose no danger. If, however, any of these are compromised, ill health is likely to follow.

Because the highly selective permeability of the intestine makes it so vulnerable to bad dietary habits and bacterial imbalances, it has developed several complex protection mechanisms. Nutrients are transported across the gut lining in one of two ways: either through the cells themselves (transcellularly) or through the gaps, or 'tight junctions', between the cells (paracellularly) as shown in the illustration.

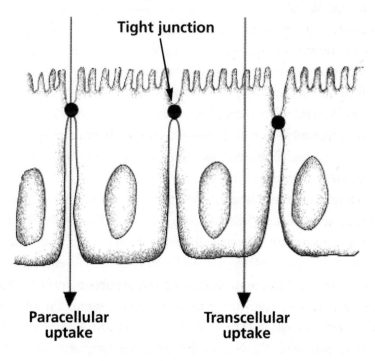

How nutrients pass across the gut lining

When either or both of these mechanisms become faulty, the gut becomes increasingly permeable, or 'leaky', allowing unwanted substances to pass across the gut wall. The gut wall is protected by intestinal secretions, which consist of, among other substances, protective mucus, immune cells that act as a benevolent police force, and secretory IgA. As we saw on page 122, this is an immunoglobulin that acts like the bouncer in a nightclub. Each SIgA molecule can remember what should or shouldn't pass into the body, and calls up immune cells to get rid of 'unwanted guests'. If SIgA levels are very low, this natural protection is lost.

What causes increased permeability?

The intestinal tract can become leaky for a number of reasons. If a person's immune system is weakened, with consequently low levels of secretory IgA (a common factor in prolonged stress) this can set the scene. Irritants to the gut lining (see Chapter 8) include gliadin in wheat,[23] excessive alcohol, coffee, tea and many other allergy-provoking foods. Any deficiency of cell-building nutrients, such as vitamin A, zinc, glutamine and essential fats, can result in a poor gut-wall structure. An overgrowth of unhealthy bacteria or fungi, such as *Candida albicans* (see Chapter 24) or any other parasite, can burrow into the intestinal wall, irritating it and causing increased permeability. Even abdominal distension, as a result of either bloating or overeating, can overstress the gut wall. Antibiotics, aspirin and other anti-inflammatory drugs are especially damaging to the gut, as we saw in Chapter 13.

The common causes of leaky gut syndrome are:

alcohol
anti-inflammatory drugs (such as aspirin)
antibiotics
chemotherapy/radiotherapy
dysbiosis (bacterial imbalance)
food allergies
gastrointestinal disease
infections (bacteria, viruses, yeasts, parasites)
inflammatory bowel disease
long-term stress
low-fibre diet
nutritional deficiencies (such as vitamin A, zinc,
    glutamine, omega-3 essential fats, and so on)
poor digestion
secretory IgA deficiency

As we have seen, increased permeability does not increase the absorption of essential nutrients. Indeed, this is likely to be reduced, as the workings of the lining are affected by damage and inflammation. Once gut permeability is increased, a vicious circle might begin, whereby the passage of toxins and undigested food particles into the body creates conditions that exacerbate the situation. Read further regarding: liver overload (see Chapter 25), malabsorption, allergy (see Chapter 10) and dysbiosis (see Chapter 14).

Leaky gut – a consequence or a cause?

Ironically, once the liver becomes increasingly overloaded with toxins, toxic chemicals can be excreted in bile and can then re-enter the digestive tract, contributing to further intestinal damage.[24] Also, the increased inflammation of the digestive tract actually stops the body from absorbing health-promoting nutrients needed by the liver and by the body to produce digestive enzymes.

It's a vicious circle in which leaky gut syndrome creates the conditions for leaky gut syndrome![25]

The link between allergies and a leaky gut is another 'chicken-and-the-egg' situation in that each can give rise to the other. Allergies might manifest in a number of ways, including eczema, fatigue and so on. Some scientists propose that food allergies contribute to leaky gut syndrome in asthmatics, for example, due to an increased allergy load overwhelming the gut's immune system.[26] Dr Leo Galland, author of The Power of Healing, suggests that chemicals such as histamine, released in response to allergens, increase permeability. A number of studies have shown that people with food allergies or intolerances have increased permeability in a fasting state, which is further exacerbated when an offending food is ingested.[27]

Dysbiosis (an imbalance of gut flora, discussed in the last chapter) is also a likely cause and consequence of leaky gut syndrome. A low level of stomach acid can also contribute, since a healthy level normally destroys microorganisms that can further damage the digestive tract. It appears that increased permeability can even lead to the gut's immune system overreacting to normal gut bacteria as well as pathogenic organisms, once again increasing permeability.

How to assess gut permeability

In view of the fact that leaky gut has been implicated in an array of health problems, restoring or ensuring the healthy condition of the intestinal lining is a key factor in improving digestive health. If you have any of the health problems listed on page 154 that have not responded to treatment, or if you score high on the list of common causes on page 157, it would be well worth finding out if you have increased intestinal permeability.

There are tests that can give a clear indication of how leaky (or permeable) the gut lining is. One test involves drinking certain chemicals that are not digested in the human body and then taking a urine sample to measure how readily they have passed through the intestinal wall. Small molecules (for example, mannitol) easily diffuse through cells, whereas larger molecules (for example, disaccharide lactulose) do not normally pass across the intestinal wall. Mannitol can therefore be used to measure absorption through cells, and lactulose acts as a marker for the integrity of the gaps between cells (the tight junctions). A gut permeability test therefore involves the ingestion of particular amounts of these two molecules in a solution. Urine gathered over the following six hours is then checked for its levels of mannitol and lactulose and compared with a pre-test sample.

High levels of lactulose in the post-ingestion urine sample show that there is increased intestinal permeability or a leaky gut, whereas low levels of mannitol indicate that malabsorption of nutrients is a problem. A nutritional therapist would be able to arrange such a test and interpret the results.

How to heal a leaky gut

Healing a leaky gut broadly involves three steps:

1. Remove the cause.
2. Improve gut flora and function.
3. Repair the gut.

In order for the cause of leaky gut to be removed, it must first be detected. Factors to consider are drugs (such as NSAIDs), alcohol, caffeine, foods to which you are intolerant (most commonly wheat and dairy products), unfriendly faecal organisms (UFOs – explained in Chapter 21), candida over-growth or dysbiosis. Any improvement in intestinal health is unlikely to be achieved while these are still present.

Meanwhile, it is essential to provide the gut with an ample supply of the nutrients needed for good health and repair, such as vitamin A, zinc, glutamine, essential fats, anti-oxidants, n-acetyl-glucosamine and fibre, as I describe below.

The presence of friendly bacteria in adequate numbers is also crucial in developing and sustaining a healthy gut. Probiotic supplements containing a range of bacteria including various lactobacilli and bifidus species can help this, especially when given alongside FOS (fructo-oligosaccharides). It is important to ensure good digestion: from proper chewing and adequate levels of stomach acid to sufficient output of digestive enzymes. Each of these may be taken as supplements.

At the same time, you should avoid suspected allergens (usually wheat, gluten and dairy products), sugar, refined car-bohydrates, saturated fat and meat; and have plenty of water and fibre, as well as water- and nutrient-dense whole foods.

Supplements

The following are worth supplementing for two to four weeks to heal a leaky gut:

L-glutamine This amino acid is the most effective promoter of healing for a leaky gut.[28] The easiest and fastest way to do this is by taking two teaspoons of L-glutamine powder, one teaspoon at night, in water, just before you go to bed, and one teaspoon on rising, waiting an hour before you eat. You do not need to do this for long – two to four weeks maximum, because the gut mucosa heal rapidly as the mucosal cells are replaced, which happens on average every two weeks.

Probiotics using a combination of *Lactobacillus* and bifido-bacteria have been shown to improve gut integrity by enhancing tight-junction stability.[29]

Vitamin C, because it is required to make collagen, which is effectively the intercellular glue. Take 1–2g daily. A very small number of people are extremely sensitive to vitamin C and will experience loose bowels on this amount. If you are one of them, experiment with how much you can take without becoming too loose and take that. Alternatively, try an ascorbate form of this vitamin.

Vitamin A, in the retinol form, which is vital for cellular growth and repair. Aim for 10,000iu/3,300mcg a day.

Vitamin D is also essential for maintaining the integrity of the gut wall.[30] It is wise to supplement 15mcg/600iu every day, as well as having 30 minutes of sun exposure a day and eating oily fish and eggs as a dietary source; however, many people are low in vitamin D and, if you are, or suspect you might be, one of them, take 50mcg/2,000iu a day for one month.

Zinc is also essential for cellular growth and repair. Take 10–20mg a day.

These nutrients should be present in a personalised sup-plement programme for maintaining general health. (See Chapter 31 to work out your own programme.)

Summary– Chapter 15

If you suspect you have leaky gut syndrome, it is best to see a nutritional therapist and have a proper test. They will advise you to:

- Stay away from alcohol, wheat and fried foods.
- Supplement digestive enzymes and probiotics.
- Take a teaspoon of glutamine powder, in water, at night before bed and one in the morning, on rising.
- Investigate food intolerances that might be aggravating your gut.
- Ensure adequate vitamins A, C and D, plus zinc, both from food and supplementation.

CHAPTER 16

Fire Belly – Resolving Gut Inflammation

I f you feel uncomfortable, not better, after meals and you experience a foggy mind, headache, body aches, sluggishness, indigestion, sleepiness and fatigue, you are probably suffering from inflammation. Many of these symptoms are not caused by the food or drink you've consumed but by your body's inflammatory reaction to them. Often, the feeling we associate with a big night out – with a three-course meal and lots of alcohol – is inflammation in action.

Inflammation lies behind just about every disease process, and especially those of the digestive system, and it is a hallmark of what I call 'internal global warming'. It is the main driver of pain, redness, bloating and swelling, although you can also be in a state of inflammation without being aware of it. If you use painkillers for anything, you are experiencing inflammation.

The word 'inflammation' also has a psychological connotation of stress, anxiety and anger and, indeed, stress hormones do have an effect on inflammatory markers. One study, for example, showed that being stressed raised inflammatory markers more than being depressed, but the worst reaction of all was the result of being cynical.[31] Cynicism reflects mental inflexibility, whereas a gradual loss of physical flexibility – for example, as found in arthritis – is also a consequence of inflammation, but in this case it is of the body and not the mind. Similarly, when we hold onto negative emotions which 'eat away' at us in the belly, perhaps producing ulcers, IBS or an inflammatory bowel condition, we can see how inflammation of both the mind and body is interlinked. Inflammation levels tend to increase with age and can certainly be argued to be one of the drivers of ageing.

But what causes inflammation and how can you reduce it? As you can see in the illustration below, inflammation is part of the body's immune-system response to circumstances that don't suit it. This could be an injury, including damaging the gut with too much alcohol or wheat gluten, an infection such as food poisoning, eating a food you're allergic or intolerant to or eating too much and hence overloading the fat cells.

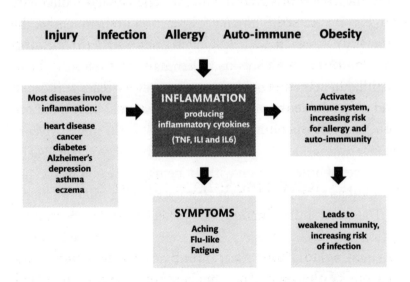

The causes and consequences of inflammation

In response to the injury, infection, allergy, autoimmune reaction or obesity, the body produces a variety of inflammatory chemicals with strange-sounding names like 'tumour necrosis factor' (TNF) and 'interleukin 6' (IL6). Scientists often measure these to find out if something is causing the inflammation. Coffee drinking, for example, increases these. These inflammation chemicals then cause the symptoms we associate with pain – aching, fatigue and flu-like symptoms. Many of the symptoms of a cold, for example, are actually produced by your immune system going into a state of inflammation, not by the virus itself. One of the best indicators of inflammation is an increase in C-reactive protein, or CRP, which goes up in response to the body being in a state of inflammation.

The higher your CRP level, the worse off you are likely to be; for example, it is a strong predictor of the severity of coronary artery disease.[32] In a study of people who had suffered a stroke, the level of CRP proved to be the best indicator of the likelihood of survival, so it is important to reduce your level if it is raised.[33] The ideal level is as low as possible, but certainly below 1mg/dl, although if you do all the right things, as described in this book, your level may well be below 0.8mg/dl, which is optimal. A level above 2.5mg/dl means roughly double the risk of cardiovascular disease. Switched-on cardiologists often measure this.

Reversing inflammation is a two-step process

According to Hippocrates, 'Illnesses do not come upon us out of the blue. They are developed from small daily sins against Nature. When enough sins have accumulated illnesses will suddenly appear.' He was certainly forward thinking, because that's exactly what today's medical science is showing.

I pay a lot of attention to factors in our diet and lifestyle that trigger an inflammatory response. These include blood sugar spikes, high insulin, coffee (but not tea to anything like the same extent), alcohol, burnt animal fats, pollution exposure, such as smoking, being in a state of stress, and eating foods you're allergic or intolerant to. Both wheat and dairy products often produce an inflammatory response. There's a vicious circle here, because once your body is in a state of inflammation and it starts to react against things, the immune system becomes over-reactive, like a belligerent police force, sometimes arresting the wrong villains. Your risk of food allergies then goes up; substances you could previously tolerate, such as air pollution, tip you into asthma; and the risk of developing autoimmune diseases that can affect the thyroid, the joints and the nerves escalates.

The illustration opposite shows the main culprits that tip you into post-meal inflammation.

Once your body begins reacting, more antibodies (designed to latch onto your allergens) float around in the bloodstream and lymphatic system. These antibodies, known as 'immunoglobulins', belong to different families, such as IgE, IgG and IgA. We investigated these in some detail in Chapter 10.

IgE antibodies are like machine guns. They instantly attack, causing immediate and severe reactions to, for example, peanuts or shellfish, if these are your triggers. I have an IgE to dairy products. Within minutes I can feel a pulsing in my nose, leading to sinus inflammation and often a migraine.

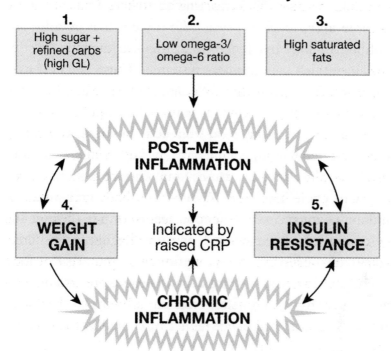

Promoters of post-meal inflammation

IgA antibodies in the gut attack invaders, such as the yeast candida. If you don't have enough of them you can end up with endemic candidiasis, an overgrowth of yeast.

IgG antibody reactions account for most food intolerances. They are like rifles compared to the machine gun of IgE, and it often takes several hours, or even up to three days, to start getting symptoms. These kinds of allergies are harder to detect by observation. Hence, my recommended first step to reducing inflammation is to remove things your immune system currently reacts against and, in the case of food or drink, the best way to find out is to have an IgG food and/or drink intolerance test (see Resources). Once you know what your immune system is reacting against you need to avoid these foods as much as possible for three to four months. IgG antibodies don't live longer than this so, theoretically, this may mean that your immune system no longer reacts against that food. Remember that the major reason we become allergic in the first place is that the wafer-thin gut membrane that separates our digesting food from our bloodstream becomes damaged, allowing incompletely digested proteins through. While you avoid your current food triggers, also heal your gut with a combination of digestive enzymes, probiotics and glutamine to reverse your food intolerances (see Chapter 17).

You will also need to avoid, or minimise, other substances or circumstances that trigger an immune response. By eating a low-GL diet, and staying away from sugar, caffeine and alcohol as much as possible, you can ease the load on your immune system, and hence reduce inflammation.

Eat more anti-inflammatory foods

Another vital step is to increase your intake of anti-inflammatory nutrients. If you do this, as well as eliminating the inflammatory triggers, you will have the maximum chance of coming out of inflammation. My favourite anti-inflammatory foods and nutrients are:

Oily fish, which is rich in omega-3 fats. It is EPA, a type of omega-3, that has the most anti-inflammatory effect.

Red onions because they are rich in quercetin, which works with vitamins C and E to protect against free-radical damage. Quercetin also has an anti-inflammatory effect by inhibiting the enzymes that produce pro-inflammatory prostaglandins. A trial in which people with rheumatoid arthritis were treated with a vegan diet, high in antioxidants including quercetin, found that they had decreased joint stiffness and pain as well as an improvement in self-reported health.[34] Quercetin also inhibits the release of histamine, which is involved in inflammatory reactions. Take 500mg quercetin per day, between meals. It becomes more bioavailable when taken with bromelain.

Bromelain, which is a collection of enzymes found in pineapples. Since it was first used in 1957, it has been shown to have a wide variety of medicinal properties – including the reduction of inflammation in rheumatoid arthritis. There are several mechanisms by which bromelain is believed to help. Firstly, it inhibits pro-inflammatory compounds and blocks the production of kinins, compounds that increase swelling and cause pain. Secondly, it helps to reduce swelling by breaking down fibrin – a mesh that forms around an inflamed area, blocking off the blood supply and impairing tissue drainage. Bromelain can be taken in supplement form: 250–750mg a day, in between meals.

Olives because they contain an extract called hydroxytyrosol, which has powerful anti-inflammatory effects. The active ingredient is a polyphenol, which has an antioxidant content over ten times greater than vitamin C. Olives also contain a compound called oleocanthal, which is chemically related to ibuprofen, although it has none of the negative side effects. In 2005 researchers at the Monell Chemical Senses Center and University of the Sciences in the US found that oleocanthal was a potent anti-inflammatory painkiller.[35]

Turmeric The bright yellow pigment of the turmeric spice contains the active compound curcumin, which has a variety of powerful anti-inflammatory actions. On top of this, it's a potent antioxidant. A review of turmeric in the *Journal of Clinical Immunology* states that curcumin at low doses can also enhance antibody responses.[36] This suggests that curcumin's reported beneficial effects in many diseases is likely to be due to its ability to modulate the immune system and reduce inflammation. You need about 500mg, one to three times a day (the equivalent of one heaped teaspoon or one capsule three times a day).

Hops contain an extract called isooxygene, one of the most potent natural inhibitors of COX-2 – an enzyme responsible for inflammation. A study compared the effects of isooxygene to ibuprofen. Two tablets of ibuprofen inhibited COX-2 by 62 per cent, while isooxygene achieved a 56 per cent inhibition.[37] Not only is isooxygene almost as effective, but it doesn't have the associated gut problems or other side effects of anti-inflammatory drugs. You need about 500–1,500mg a day.

Ginger is an effective anti-inflammatory favoured by Ayurvedic medicine. Twentieth-century technology has demonstrated that ginger inhibits the synthesis of pro-inflammatory prostaglandins and thromboxanes, another type of inflammatory mediator. Ginger also has antioxidant properties and contains an enzyme that may have a similar action to bromelain. Taking a supplement of 500–2,000mg of ginger a day is ideal. Otherwise, incorporate a 1cm slice of fresh ginger into your daily diet. If you have a juicer, make a whole glass full of ginger juice then put the juice into an ice cube tray and freeze. This gives you fresh ginger ice cubes, which you can add to hot and cold drinks and soups to give you a high-potency ginger boost.

MSM, which stands for methylsulfonylmethane, is a source of the essential mineral sulphur. Sulphur is involved in a multitude of key body functions, including pain control, detoxification and tissue building. MSM is a fantastic anti-inflammatory, but bear in mind that there are some people it does not suit. If you suffer with digestive discomfort after taking MSM, it's not for you. The therapeutic dose appears to be 1,500–3,000mg a day.

By making many of these foods a staple part of your diet, you will reduce inflammation. My kedgeree recipe (see page 366), made with mackerel and red onions, uses turmeric and olive oil to give you a good helping of natural anti-inflammatories. You can add more olives. That, and a ginger tea, is a recipe for reducing gut pain and inflammation.

Good anti-inflammatory supplements use highly concentrated combinations of these natural anti-inflammatories at doses beyond that which you can eat; for example, you can supplement 500mg of quercetin, whereas a red onion provides only 20mg. These kinds of levels are great for switching your immune system out of inflammation, but they are not necessary (although not harmful) on a daily basis if you are otherwise healthy. Together with a low-GL diet that is high in antioxidants, adopting a positive attitude and reducing your stress levels, you can switch off the fire in your belly and feel better, not worse, after meals.

This approach is the cornerstone to solving inflammatory bowel diseases such as Crohn's and ulcerative colitis, which I will explore in more detail in Chapter 19.

Summary – Chapter 16

To enhance and protect your immunity and help your body fight against pathogenic triggers:

- Have an IgG food intolerance test and avoid the foods you react to for 3–4 months.
- Supplement with digestive enzymes, probiotics and glutamine to combat food intolerances and restore gut integrity.
- Adhere to a low-GL diet which contains a minimum amount of sugar, caffeine and alcohol and is antioxidant-rich.
- Increase consumption of anti-inflammatory foods including oily fish, red onions, olives, turmeric and ginger.
- If in need, consider supplementing with optimum doses of quercetin, curcumin, hops, and MSM in combination.

CHAPTER 17

Stopping GERD and Acid Reflux

A lot of older people complain of 'acid reflux' or a burning in the chest, moving up to the throat. If they go to their GP, they are likely to be diagnosed with GERD and prescribed a drug known as a proton-pump inhibitor, or PPI, usually ending in '-prazole'. These drugs are being handed out like sweets to just about anyone who mentions the word 'indigestion' or 'heartburn'. They are officially licensed for the treatment of ulcers and for gastro-oesophageal reflux disease, or GERD.

PPI drugs work by suppressing the formation of stomach acid (betaine hydrochloride), which is absolutely vital for digesting protein into amino acids, killing off harmful bacteria in food, and absorbing vitamin B_{12}. As we saw in Chapter 4, they don't address the underlying causes of indigestion, heartburn or GERD, which is not an excess of stomach acid.

Most people's problem is caused by a weakness in the circular valve or muscle that separates the stomach from the oesophagus, called the LES (lower (o)esophageal-stomach valve). In an extreme form, this is called a hiatus hernia (see page 33). As a consequence, acid, which is meant to be contained within the stomach, passes up into the oesophagus. By simply suppressing all stomach-acid formation, you can get temporary relief, but at some quite considerable cost, as I explained in Chapter 13. After all, the body doesn't produce stomach acid for no reason.

At this point you may be thinking that if most people who have GERD have a *lack* of stomach acid, why do the drugs help? This is because if you are regurgitating stomach juices past the LES valve, even the tiniest amount of acid will produce symptoms. Killing off *all* stomach acid is like using a hammer to crack a nut, but it actually doesn't address the true cause at all.

Also, the less stomach acid you have, the less your body can kill off harmful bacteria, which then feed off undigested food and give you gas and bloating.

As we saw on page 30, it is a fact that the older you are the greater your chance will be of having low levels of stomach acid. Stomach acid secretion declines by about 20 per cent per decade from the age of 30. Because vitamin B_{12} requires intrinsic factor, which is produced in a healthy stomach producing sufficient acid, two in five people over 60 have insufficient B_{12} in their blood – not from dietary deficiency but from poor absorption caused by a lack of stomach-acid secretions. The fact that GERD almost only develops in older people illustrates that the problem isn't caused by an excess of stomach acid, so taking antacids will never cure the problem. So what does?

What makes the lower oesophageal-stomach (LES) valve weak?

If you eat too much, this puts pressure on the valve, as does being overweight (because there is less space for the stomach). Also, if you eat too many carbs and sugary foods, which bacteria feed off, thereby producing gas, that makes matters worse. Furthermore, if you overeat protein, which stimulates more acid secretions, that can make the problem worse – as can too much coffee and alcohol, both of which are digestive irritants.

To begin with, if you eat according to my low-GL principles, which I explain in Chapter 32, you will avoid these problems. If you also take, with each main meal, a digestive-support supplement that contains both digestive enzymes and beneficial bacteria, you will take a load off your stomach and help prevent the formation of gas and the pressure it creates. Some of these digestive-support supplements also contain some glutamine, which helps keep the lining of the digestive tract healthy.

Watch out for too much coffee (I recommend just one at the start of the day, away from food, if you feel you have to) and alcohol (one drink maximum a day and if possible none during the week). Also, don't lie down after meals. Stay upright.

One common reason for heartburn is eating food you are allergic or intolerant to. Babies, when given cow's milk too early, regurgitate it. This normal reflux is what the body does to get rid of something that doesn't suit it. If you keep eating the wrong foods, this can weaken the circular muscle at the top of the stomach until some stomach acid enters the oesophagus, producing symptoms of heartburn. Other things that aggravate the digestive tract include NSAID painkillers (aspirin and ibuprofen), which should be avoided if you have indigestion. But most important is to test for food allergies or intolerances. (See Resources.)

High-protein foods such as meat require a greater release of stomach acid, so serve yourself smaller portions. High-protein diets, for this reason, can be aggravating for some people.

Another possible cause of digestive pain is the presence of stomach ulcers, often caused by infection with *Helicobacter pylori* (see Chapter 18 for more details on this). Other gut infections from bacteria, yeasts (see Chapter 24) or parasites (see Chapter 21) can cause digestive symptoms. If you have followed all the advice given here, this is an avenue worth exploring, especially if your problems started after a trip abroad in a 'high-risk' region for parasites.

Are you deficient in stomach acid?

If you are older and suffering from GERD, the chances are that you are low in stomach acid. The production of stomach acid is dependent on zinc, and without enough of it you can't break proteins down properly. Make sure you are supplementing 10–20mg of zinc a day. A good multivitamin–mineral taken twice a day could give you this, but do check the label first.

Some people lack stomach acid and benefit from supplementing betaine hydrochloride (called betaine HCl – betaine is also known as trimethylglycine or TMG). This is usually bought in 300mg or 600mg strength, and relief for indigestion can be obtained by taking between 600mg and 3,000mg; however, you might want to do this under the guidance of a nutritional therapist. (TMG is also present in some homocysteine-lowering formulas as, together with zinc, it effectively lowers homocysteine and improves methylation, vital for making stomach acid, enzymes and many gut-related processes from absorption to detoxification.)

Firstly, if you don't need betaine hydrochloride, don't take it. It could make you feel worse, giving you a burning sensation. Secondly, only ever take betaine hydrochloride with a meal containing protein. Thirdly, never take it if you are on

NSAID painkillers such as aspirin or ibuprofen. As we have seen, these drugs can, and do, damage the gut, and if you have any damage or ulceration, taking betaine hydrochloride will make you worse. However, if you suffer from continuous indigestion, bloating and other problems associated with a lack of betaine hydrochloride, keep taking it, doubling the dose with each protein meal up to 3,000mg to see if you get relief. If you don't, or if you have adverse symptoms, stop taking it.

Summary – Chapter 17

Rather than suppressing the symptoms by taking antacids with considerable long-term adverse effects, try:

- Eating smaller meals, with a balance of 20 per cent protein, 30 per cent fat and 50 per cent low-GL carbohydrates, as given in my recipes.
- Test for, and avoid, foods to which you are intolerant.
- Minimise your use of coffee and alcohol.
- Take a digestive-support supplement that provides both beneficial bacteria and digestive enzymes, possibly also with glutamine, with each main meal.
- Control your weight.
- Don't lie down after eating.
- If you are still suffering, do get checked for stomach ulcers, often caused by *Helicobacter pylori* infection.
- If you've done all this and you don't have stomach ulcers, also try supplementing betaine HCl bearing in mind the cautions listed above.

CHAPTER 18

Solving Stomach Ulcers

M ost, but not all, stomach ulcers are caused, in part, by infection by the bacterium *Helicobacter pylori*. If you think that you might have an ulcer, the first step is to get your doctor to check if you have the bacterium. Conventionally, ulcers are treated with a combination of two antibiotics, plus a proton-pump inhibitor (PPI) drug, which stops you making stomach acid. But there are natural remedies that work.

PPI drugs should be for short-term use only, as the suppression of stomach acid is extremely bad for nutrient absorption and leads to all sorts of complications as a result, including the increased risk of osteoporosis, brain shrinkage and infections (see page 139).

There is plenty you can do nutritionally, however, to prevent stomach ulcers and to help them heal, rather than simply relieving the symptoms.

Before I show you what to do, it is important to understand that ulcers can manifest from other 'perfect storms', hitting the stomach (peptic ulcer) or duodenum (duodenal ulcer). These include prolonged stress, which shuts down digestion; use of painkillers, which damage the intestinal wall; overuse of caffeine, which irritates the intestinal wall; lack of key nutrients such as vitamins A and C, and zinc; dysbiosis, perhaps following antibiotic use; excessive daily consumption of alcohol; and daily consumption of foods to which you are intolerant. It is hardly surprising, then, that a combination of such factors would 'rot' the gut and create the circumstances where a harmful bacteria such as *H. pylori* can thrive. How to eliminate these factors and calm down the gut has already been explained in Chapter 16, which focuses on resolving gut inflammation.

Natural remedies that help treat *H. pylori* infection

Probiotics (beneficial bacteria) – *Acidophilus* and *Bifidus* bacteria – slow the growth of *H. pylori* in six weeks[38] and can even kill it. Probiotics can also significantly reduce the side effects and improve the effectiveness of conventional treatment. I recommend taking a high-strength probiotic providing 10 billion CFUs daily a week before, and for three months after, antibiotic therapy. (Probiotics are graded by the number of colony-forming units (CFUs) contained in them – it's a way of saying 'live and healthy microbes'.)

Oregano is one of the best natural agents against *H. pylori*, and it is thought to work by inhibiting the way *H. pylori* produces chemicals that neutralise acid in their vicinity, allowing them to survive, so it is effectively a natural antibiotic. You can buy capsules or tinctures. Take 15–45mg a day.

Deglycyrrhised liquorice root (DGL) also suppresses *H. pylori* growth and helps to repair and strengthen the stomach lining. Take 500–1,500mg a day. Make sure you take the DGL form, since liquorice can raise blood pressure if taken in the long term.

Mastic gum is another remedy that's making headlines, although the evidence is not conclusive. It has been used in traditional Greek medicine for thousands of years for various gastrointestinal disorders, including peptic ulcers. Researchers in Greece in 2012 found that although it did not completely eradicate *H. pylori*, it reduced numbers.[39] It's worth trying, although it's not proven to have no side effects. Take 1,000mg twice a day for three months.

I would recommend taking probiotics before having the usual triple therapy (which is two antibiotics, plus a PPI drug, as mentioned above), then having the triple therapy followed by natural remedies for three months under the guidance of a nutritional therapist.

How to reduce acid-stimulating foods and gastric irritants

The stomach produces acid to digest protein. Following a high-protein diet (high in meat, fish and eggs) is likely to aggravate inflamed stomach membranes further.

Coffee and alcohol, as well as non-steroidal anti-inflammatory painkillers (NSAIDs) also aggravate the gut wall. The combination of painkillers and alcohol, if you have ulceration, is extremely dangerous, as it can cause internal bleeding.

Nevertheless, oily fish has the advantage of containing anti-inflammatory omega-3 fats, which help to calm down inflamed membranes, so eating oily fish in moderation is likely to do more good than harm.

Although spicy foods are thought to be acid forming, in fact they are alkaline and, provided you don't feel worse, evidence shows that they don't make ulcers worse. They are, however, quite high up on the list of the most common foods provoking intolerances, so they don't suit everyone.

Heal the gut with vitamin A and glutamine

Vitamin A and the amino acid glutamine help to regenerate healthy epithelial cells, which line the digestive tract. Glutamine is best taken as a powder: take 1 heaped teaspoon (5g) in a glass of cold water last thing at night on an empty stomach. A generous supply of glutamine can help repair and maintain a healthy small-intestinal lining. Taking this for a month can help to heal ulcers.

Vitamin A, in the animal form called retinol, is also vital for healthy cells in the stomach. Although high doses are not recommended during pregnancy, if you are unlikely to become pregnant, or if you are male, taking high doses for a month can help to speed up the healing of ulcers.

Vitamin C also helps healing, but too much, especially in the slightly acid ascorbic-acid form, can aggravate ulcers. Either limit your intake to 200mg or take an alkaline form of vitamin C such as a mineral ascorbate.

Although there are no human trials to date, animals with gastric ulcers have been helped by taking sea buckthorn, a rich source of omega-7 fats.[40] You might gain further benefits from supplementing sea buckthorn, as it also contains other ulcer-repairing antioxidant and anti-inflammatory substances, including carotenoids, vitamin E and omegas-3, -6 and -9.

Check for, and avoid, allergens and foods to which you are intolerant

Eating any food you are allergic to, or intolerant of, will increase inflammation and aggravate an ulcer. An unidentified food allergy might even precipitate this condition, especially if you have undiagnosed celiac disease (see Chapter 20).

What to eat to reduce your risk of stomach ulcers

The best foods to eat to reduce your risk of stomach ulcers are low-allergenic and high in nutrients: for example, vegetables, non-citrus fruits, oats, red onions, garlic, quinoa and oily fish. The worst foods are alcohol, meat, dairy and coffee.

Supplementary benefit

In terms of supplements, I recommend:

2 × high-potency multivitamin–minerals with at least 5mcg of B_{12} and 10mg of zinc, plus 200mg of vitamin C – this should not be too much to aggravate an ulcer, especially if in an ascorbate form.

1–2 × essential omegas with fish-oil-derived omega-3, plus omega-6 from borage or evening primrose oil. Omega-3 particularly calms down gut inflammation.

3 × vitamin A 5,000iu capsules (5,000mcg in total) in the retinol form. An alternative would be cod liver oil capsules. Some are high in omega-3, vitamin D and vitamin A.

1 × digestive enzyme supplement with each main meal.

2 × probiotic supplements giving a total of 5–10 billion viable organisms a day.

1 teaspoon (5g) glutamine powder in water last thing at night on an empty stomach.

Or
3 × combined digestive enzyme, probiotic and glutamine formula (these rarely give enough glutamine and may not supply enough probiotics for serious gut healing, so they might be better taken after two weeks for maintenance of a gut-healing programme).

Optional
2 × omega-7 (sea buckthorn oil) 250mg.

If you have *Helicobacter pylori* infection, follow the guidelines above in relation to supplements.

CAUTIONS Vitamin C, although good for general health, can further aggravate a stomach ulcer. It is better to limit your intake to 200mg until your ulcers are healed.

Summary – Chapter 18

To eliminate the risk of developing stomach ulcers as well as alleviating existing ones, I suggest the following:

- Check with your GP if you are infected with *Helicobacter pylori*, as this bacterium is the predominant underlying cause of digestive pain and stomach ulcers.
- Avoid allergenic and gastric irritants, as well as foods you know you are intolerant to, to avoid inflammation.
- To prevent microbial growth, try either of the natural remedies mentioned above: a potent probiotic that contains *Acidophilus* and Bifidus bacteria, mastic gum for 3 months or DGL. Alternatively, sea buckthorn will provide you with antioxidant and anti-inflammatory properties for gut healing.
- Consume nutrient-rich foods that have low allergenic potential: vegetables, non-citrus fruits, oats, red onions, garlic, quinoa and oily fish. If you are not intolerant, try spicy foods to neutralise induced acidity from foods.
- Supplement with multivitamin–minerals that contain B_{12}, zinc and vitamin C, essential omegas-3 and -6, vitamin A in its retinol or cod liver oil forms, and a limited amount of 200mg of vitamin C in either its alkaline or mineral ascorbate forms.
- Supplement with digestive enzymes, probiotics and glutamine on their own or in a combination formula.

CHAPTER 19

Conquering Crohn's, Ulcerative Colitis and Inflammatory Bowel Disease

Unlike the broader and more hazy 'diagnosis' of irritable bowel syndrome, Crohn's and ulcerative colitis are inflammatory bowel diseases that can be positively diagnosed by the presence of inflammation along the digestive tract. Although the advice for irritable bowel syndrome (IBS) is relevant to these cases too, the emphasis in correcting Crohn's and ulcerative colitis should be on removing the causes of inflammation, reducing the inflammation itself and healing the digestive tract. If you suffer from ulcerative colitis, see also page 283 for advice on colitis, which is often the precursor to this condition.

Crohn's and ulcerative colitis are the two major types of what is known as inflammatory bowel disease (IBD). They are much more complex than the conditions we have so far discussed in the book, involving abnormal immune-system responses, possibly allergies, intestinal permeability and genetic factors. Crohn's and ulcerative colitis now affect one in every 1,000 people and, without proper treatment, can necessitate surgery to remove the damaged section of the digestive tract.

Whether a person is diagnosed with Crohn's or ulcerative colitis depends on the location and type of inflammation, as well as the symptoms. Ulcerative colitis causes inflammation of the lining of the colon only. Classic symptoms are passing blood and mucus, pain before defecation, a general feeling of tiredness and, in more severe cases, diarrhoea. Crohn's disease can affect any part of the bowel, usually the last part of the small intestine (the ileum), in a more severe way, thickening the intestinal wall, although often the bowel is normal in between the inflamed sections.

Inflammatory bowel disease – a complex equation

Although there is no one universal therapy for inflammatory bowel disease, a complex picture is emerging of a number of causative factors which together lead to inflammation of the bowel. These factors include:

- A genetically inherited tendency towards inflammation.
- Certain food allergies or sensitivities.
- Dysbiosis (see Chapter 14), including bacterial imbalance and infections.
- Increased intestinal permeability.
- Detoxification problems.

In a study of children in the Newcastle area of the UK, researchers from the Royal Victoria Infirmary found that those with

Crohn's disease had a six-fold increase in intestinal permeability.[41] In another study at St Bartholomew's Hospital in London, children with Crohn's disease and intestinal permeability were fed a diet of pure nutrients (not food as such) for six weeks. As a consequence, there was both a substantial improvement in their symptoms and in their intestinal permeability.[42] Indeed, many researchers have found that low-allergenic diets can produce significant relief both from Crohn's and ulcerative colitis. The most common offending foods are wheat, milk and yeast, although the ideal diet varies from person to person.

The first step in its correction is therefore to identify the offending foods and eliminate them. The next step is to correct dysbiosis and re-inoculate the digestive tract with the correct beneficial bacteria. There is some evidence that the wrong balance of bacteria might generate toxins that then damage the intestinal wall. The wrong bacterial imbalance can also affect immune function, leading to increased inflammation in the digestive tract, so balancing this is important.

The amino acid glutamine is especially important in healing the digestive tract. The main medical treatment, however, is the use of anti-inflammatory drugs to calm down the inflammation, or medication to turn off the body's immune reactions. These drugs are effective but they do nothing to address the actual causes of the inflammation. According to Dr Jeffrey Bland, a pioneer in new approaches to inflammation, 'Instead of thinking "pain means drug", inflammation is the body's way of saying something is wrong. Inflammation is a "systemic" problem, not just a localised phenomenon, in which the body's physiology is shifted into an "alarm" state.' It's as if there is a series of underlying imbalances in the body's chemistry that build up and then burst forth when the body can no longer cope with a set of circumstances. The actual pain is the wave breaking, although the wave is a long time coming. From this perspective, there are several factors that set the scene for inflammation, and then those that trigger the manifestation of symptoms.

The inflammatory process

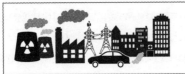

ENVIRONMENT
Allergens, toxins, stress, infections, trauma, lowered oxygen, drugs, alcohol

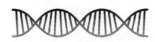

GENES
Many possible expressions, including inherited susceptibilities

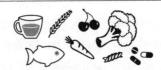

DIET
Macronutrients, micronutrients, accessory nutrients, phytonutrients

FUNCTION
Shifts physiological state into 'alarm' reaction characterised by inflammatory process

SYMPTOMS OF INFLAMMATION
-osis becomes -itis with increasing severity

So often, it's the 'hair that broke the camel's back' that gets the blame. You often hear reasons like 'My colitis started when my marriage was breaking up' or 'Ever since I had that bout of flu I started to get abdominal pain.' These triggers are important and may include a trauma, an allergy, an infection, a toxin or exposure to too many oxidants.

One would hope that a healthy person could rise to such challenges, but if there are underlying weaknesses, such as a genetic predisposition or poor nutritional status, the person might have no reserves in their 'health bank'. In this case, the slightest stress might tip them over into an inflammatory state. If this persists, the immune system gets hyper-reactive and can switch over into a belligerent state that attacks the gut. This is called autoimmunity.

Switching off autoimmunity

Your immune system is designed to react to unwelcome substances from the outside world, such as viruses, harmful bacteria, pathogens and food allergens, and also to misbehaving cells such as cancer cells. But sometimes the immune system can also attack healthy cells. This results in autoimmune diseases such as Crohn's and ulcerative colitis.

Wrongly, many people think that since the immune system seems to be overreacting, anything that could boost the immune system – for example, vitamin C – could make matters worse. But autoimmune diseases are a 'system-control' problem, and many of the foods and nutrients that help an immune system to work make matters *better* not worse.

Celiac disease, an extreme form of wheat allergy that I discuss fully in Chapter 20, is very common among sufferers of Crohn's and ulcerative colitis, and it should always be screened for. As we saw earlier, celiac disease is an extreme reaction to gluten, and usually the gliadin protein, which is present in wheat, rye and barley, but not in oats.

It is also important to find out if the body is producing IgG antibodies or IgE antibodies, indicating intolerance to certain foods. (See Chapter 10 to find out how to test for and eliminate allergies.) The theory is that if the immune system becomes hyper-alert against foods, it cross-reacts against certain body tissues. The goal, therefore, is to eliminate the food and lessen the immune system's belligerent attitude.

What is interesting is that 80 per cent of celiac sufferers don't react to oats, which are not only gliadin-free but also a rich source of beta-glucans. Beta-glucans, which are especially rich in oat fibre, might help to lessen autoimmunity and improve general health in a counter-intuitive way. One of the prevalent theories as to why autoimmune diseases are on the increase is that we live in environments that are too clean and we don't get enough exposure to early bugs and bacteria. Most such microbes have beta-glucans present in their cell walls, and beta-glucans consequently stimulate the immune system and help to build up normal, strong immunity. Many known immune enhancers – from shiitake mushrooms to echinacea – are rich sources of beta-glucans. Beta-glucans appears to act as an immune-system modulator and might also help autoimmune diseases. As well as eating more oats and shiitake mushrooms, you can buy supplements of purified beta-glucans. Choose those that contain (1–3)(1–6) beta-d-glucans.

Another potential trigger for autoimmunity is sugar, because having too high sugar levels leads to proteins in the body being damaged, called glycosylation, in such a way that they might start to misbehave, or no longer be recognised as friend, but rather foe, by the body's immune system. These damaged proteins are called AGEs (advanced glycation end-products) and the more you have the more your immune system is likely to react. Particularly bad is fructose (fruit sugar), which the body finds harder to burn, or turn directly into fat, than glucose. If you follow my low-GL diet, you will naturally be limiting your fructose intake to healthy levels. (For more information, see *The Low-GL Diet Bible* or *The Low-GL Diet Cookbook*, or read the section on low-GL eating on my website: www.patrickholford.com.)

Another successful diet approach to autoimmune diseases is a Paleo diet, or a Stone Age diet. Before we became peasant farmers, so to speak, humans lived on meat from fit and wild animals – not factory-farmed animals – plus seafood, plants, fruit and nuts. We weren't yet eating grains or dairy products. Many people with autoimmune diseases today report great improvements eating an essentially grain- and dairy-free diet.

Another difference between modern living and Paleo living would have been vitamin D exposure. Given that we are originally designed to be naked, outdoors and living in Africa, our exposure to vitamin D, primarily made in the skin in the presence of sunlight, but also found in oily fish, has drastically declined. Vitamin D deficiency is linked to an increasing risk of autoimmune diseases. We need at least 30mcg a day, and eating oily fish and exposing a decent part of yourself to 30 minutes of sunlight might give you 15mcg, so it's best to supplement at least another 15mcg a day.

Inflammatory bowel diseases are also increasingly prevalent in regions further away from the equator (and hence the sunlight) and sufferers do often have low vitamin D levels, which should, ideally, be above 75ng/ml. Although the evidence is limited at the moment, generally showing benefit for Crohn's but not for ulcerative colitis, there is growing evidence that higher amounts, 50–250mcg/2,000–10,000iu a day, might help switch off autoimmunity.[43]

Healing the gut

Studies show that those with Crohn's disease have increased gut permeability, which thereby increases the chance of developing allergies. This is because food proteins cross through the gut wall and the immune system reacts against them. Eating a highly nutritious diet, with low-allergenic foods, will help to both health the gut and lessen symptoms. As we have seen, the most common offending foods are wheat, milk and yeast, although the ideal diet will vary from person to person.

The first step in the correction of Crohn's and ulcerative colitis therefore lies in identifying the offending foods and eliminating them. (See Chapter 10.)

The next step is to correct dysbiosis and to re-inoculate the digestive tract with the right beneficial bacteria. There is some evidence that the wrong balance of bacteria might generate toxins that then damage the intestinal wall. The wrong bacterial imbalance can also affect immune function leading to increased inflammation in the digestive tract, so balancing this is important. Although I would still recommend a probiotic supplement providing both *Lactobacillus* and bifidobacteria, studies giving these to IBD sufferers have shown little benefit to date. It is worth testing to find out if you have SIBO (small intestinal bacterial overgrowth), in which case probiotics are more likely to help. A nutritional therapist can do this for you by arranging for you to have a methane/hydrogen breath test.

A low-FODMAP diet (see page 241) which aims to eliminate all foods, including prebiotics, that feed bacteria is quite often helpful for those with inflammatory bowel disease.[44]

The amino acid glutamine is especially important in healing the digestive tract, because the epithelial cells that make up the gut wall are regenerated by it. Look for supplements that combine digestive enzymes with probiotics and glutamine, but also take a teaspoon of glutamine powder (about 5g), in water last thing at night to accelerate gut healing.

Increase nature's anti-inflammatories

As we saw earlier in this chapter, the main medical treatment for any inflammatory bowel disease is the use of anti-inflammatory drugs to actually calm down the inflammation or medication to turn off the body's immune reactions. Inflammation is the body's way of saying something is wrong. It is a systemic problem, not just a localised phenomenon, in which the body's physiology is shifted into an alarm state. Just taking anti-inflammatory drugs fails to address the underlying causes.

While there are several factors that set the scene for inflammation, there are also those that trigger the manifestation of symptoms. These triggers are important and might include a trauma, an allergy, an infection, a toxin or exposure to too many oxidants. All these factors need to be considered to restore health.

A diet high in meat and milk, which are rich sources of the pro-inflammatory fat arachidonic acid, encourages inflammation. In contrast, a diet high in omega-3 fats, found in flax and chia seeds and oily fish, switches off inflammation. (If using flax seeds, make sure you grind them or soak them overnight to avoid any potential for gut irritation. This is not so necessary with chia, although it might help those with a really sensitive digestive system.)

Fish oils, high in the omega-3 family of fats, and particularly EPA, are well known for fighting inflammation. Most inflammatory disease responds best to about 1,000mg of EPA. This means taking two high-strength omega-3 fish oil capsules a day.

There are also a number of natural anti-inflammatory agents found in common foods. These include:

Turmeric Curcumin, the active ingredient in the yellow curry spice turmeric, works as well as anti-inflammatory drugs, but without the side effects.

Olive extracts The first is hydroxytyrosol – a very powerful antioxidant with anti-inflammatory effects. This is a polyphenol, a type of compound found in foods that has positive health effects. Another key ingredient is oleocanthal, which is chemically related to ibuprofen, although it has none of the negative side effects. Studies on olive pulp extract have shown that it reduces the levels of two inflammatory messengers called TNF-alpha and interleukin-8.

Hop extract An extract from hops, called isooxygene, is one of the most potent natural COX-2 inhibitors, which is the enzyme many painkillers block, and one of the most effective natural painkillers of all. It works just as well as painkilling drugs but it doesn't cause gut damage.

Quercetin This is a potent anti-inflammatory found in red onions. One red onion, or a cup of berries, or three servings of greens provides about 20mg of quercetin. However, at 25 times this amount, 500mg a day, quercetin becomes a potent anti-inflammatory, inhibiting the production of the pro-inflammatory prostaglandins (type-2) and also inhibiting the release of histamine, which is involved in inflammatory reactions.

Look for supplements containing concentrates of these natural anti-inflammatory agents.

Choose soluble fibres

Crohn's and colitis sufferers are rightly wary of eating high-fibre food, which can irritate the gut, and are often advised to avoid fibre to help heal the gut. But soluble fibres are different. These are found in foods such as oats, chia and flax seeds, and they absorb water and partially dissolve, as in porridge. These soluble fibres are much more gentle on the digestive tract and help to move faecal matter along, which is essential for gut health. If you grind and/or soak oats, flax or chia seeds, or saturate them in water, as in porridge, all the better. Oats are a rich source of beta-glucans, which, as we have seen, are beneficial to health.

Improve your methylation

One of the key 'control' mechanisms of the body is methylation. It's a chemical process that is needed for just about everything in your body: producing energy, building bones and joints, neurotransmitters and hormones, as well as detoxifying, repairing DNA and copying the correct information to make new cells. There are a billion methylation reactions taking place in nearly every cell in your body and brain every few seconds. Methylation is dependent on B vitamins and other methyl nutrients to work optimally. It is therefore not surprising to find that people with autoimmune diseases are much more likely to be deficient in the B vitamins, which manifests in a raised homocysteine level, which is the best indicator of poor methylation. This can be easily tested using a home-test kit. If your homocysteine level is high, there are specific nutrients (B_2, B_6, B_{12}, folic acid, TMG, NAC and zinc) that you need to take in specific amounts to normalise your level. The correct amount to take, depending on your homocysteine level, is explained in a report that I have prepared on my website. (See Resources.)

The best and worst foods

The best foods to eat for all forms of IBD are oily fish (such as salmon, mackerel, herring and sardines), ground and soaked chia seeds, soaked oats – as in porridge (use soft oats) – berries and soft fruits, steamed vegetables, rice (white during the healing phase) and quinoa. You also might want to test how you react to the ancient wheat, Kamut khorasan (see page 92), which has been shown to have anti-inflammatory effects, unlike modern wheat.

The worst foods are sugar, wheat, dairy products, yeast and those high in insoluble fibres, such as wheat bran.

Supplementary benefit

I recommend taking these daily for all forms of IBD:

2 × vitamin C 1,000mg

2 × vitamin D drops (25mcg) – for up to 3 months

2 × (1–3)(1–6) beta-d-glucans

1 × combination supplement with digestive enzymes, probiotics and glutamine with each meal

2 × omega-3-rich fish oil to achieve 1,000mg of EPA

1 teaspoon (5g) glutamine powder in water last thing at night on an empty stomach for 1 month.

3 × combination formula providing turmeric (curcumin), olive and hop extracts, and quercetin

CAUTIONS: Although high-fibre foods are good for digestion during the healing phase, be wary of including too much whole grains, nuts, seeds and raw vegetables. If foods are ground, soaked or steamed, some of the plant fibres break down and become gentler on the digestive tract.

Summary – Chapter 19

To attenuate all forms of IBD and correct autoimmunity:

- Identify foods you are allergic or intolerant to, to eliminate inflammatory triggers.
- Consume rich sources of beta-glucans from shiitake mushrooms, oats or in purified supplement form.
- Follow my steps to a low-GL diet.
- It would be best to keep sugar, specifically fructose, wheat, dairy and yeast consumption to a minimum and consider adhering to the Paleo diet.
- Favour a diet rich in oily fish (salmon, mackerel, herring, sardines), ground and soaked oats, flax and chia seeds or in EPA-enriched fish oils to obtain an adequate amount of your essential omega-3s. Rice, quinoa and Kamut khorasan may also help fight inflammation.
- Consider adopting a diet rich in turmeric, hop and olive extracts and red onions or the potent anti-inflammatory agents that are found in these foods in a combined supplement formula.
- Consider supplementing probiotics that contain *Lactobacillus* and bifidobacteria, particularly if you have SIBO. Alternatively, you may also supplement these in a combined formula with digestive enzymes and glutamine at meal times.
- Monitor your homocysteine levels to identify whether you need to supplement B vitamins.
- Recommended supplements include 1,000mg vitamin C, 25mcg vitamin D for 3 months and beta-d-glucans.

CHAPTER 20

Diagnosing and Coping with Celiac Disease

C eliac disease is a permanent disease of the small
intestine, caused by an allergic toxicity to the gliadin
protein found in gluten cereals. Where the condition
is present, the lining of the small intestine is relentlessly
attacked by the gliadin (it doesn't take much – less than 0.5g a
day can cause this reaction). The lining becomes damaged and
loses its ability to absorb nutrients from food. Malabsorption
and malnutrition therefore follow, inducing deficiencies in
iron, zinc, calcium, magnesium, potassium and vitamins B_6,
B_{12}, folic acid and vitamins A, D, E and K.

There is a strong genetic component in celiac disease. In
identical twins, for example, of those who suffer, in 70 per
cent of cases both twins will have it, making it 175 times more
prevalent among twins than the general population. If you
have a mother, father, brother or sister with celiac disease, you
have a one in ten chance of having it too, which means you
have a 30 times higher risk than the average person.

Many medical textbooks still say, wrongly, that it occurs
in only one in five thousand or so people. Due to remarkable

advancements in laboratory screening for celiac disease, however, we have learnt that it occurs more frequently than ever imagined. As I explained in Chapter 9, one in ten celiac sufferers go undiagnosed. Of those with digestive problems, about one in 40 children and one in 30 adults have celiac disease, although few are diagnosed as such.[45]

Celiac disease is thought to be such a health threat in Italy that the Italian government recommends that all children be tested for gliadin sensitivity and celiac disease by the age of six. Things are, however, rather different in the UK, where GPs rarely check for celiac disease.

Screening and diagnosing celiac disease

Celiac disease used to be diagnosed by means of a gut biopsy showing atrophy (damage) of the intestinal villi (the cells that line the intestine). It is commonly an outpatient procedure performed by a specialist, and involves a long tube being inserted through the mouth, oesophagus, stomach and finally into the small intestine, where several biopsies of mucosal lining are taken. A pathologist, looking for the characteristic mucosal lesions of celiac disease, then studies these small pieces of tissue under a microscope.

Although a gut biopsy is certainly thorough, it is also expensive and inconvenient. Many doctors and their patients are understandably reluctant to have it performed unless there is very good reason for doing so. This is where modern laboratory science comes into play.

Several antibody blood tests are currently being used with great success to help distinguish people who are likely candidates for celiac disease from those who aren't. People with a positive screening now have a greater incentive to have a biopsy performed, with a much higher percentage of biopsies then coming back positive for celiac disease. At the same time, fewer unnecessary and costly biopsies are performed.

Gliadin – The main culprit

Since gliadin appears to be the key offending protein to which celiac sufferers are reacting, testing whether you are producing antibodies to gliadin is a useful place to start. Often, people with celiac disease produce anti-gliadin IgA antibodies, along with anti-gliadin IgG antibodies. When you have an IgG food intolerance test, one of the hundred or so foods you'll be tested for will be gliadin, so you'll get this information with your results.

There is a problem with relying on just an IgG gliadin test, however. If you don't have celiac disease, you can still test positive. You might be gliadin sensitive, but not have celiac disease. Also, if you've strictly avoided all sources of gluten/gliadin for several months, you might not test positive.

The answer to the dilemma is a test called IgA anti-transglutaminase (IgA-TGA). This is the newest lab test for celiac disease. It measures anti-transglutaminase, which is a key enzyme that is targeted when you have celiac disease. In a recent study all celiac sufferers (100 per cent) were found to react positively to this test, and also the greater the level of reactivity, the greater was the level of damage to gut mucosa.[46] The test, therefore, not only tested whether or not the person was sensitive, but also the degree of sensitivity.

If you test and your result is positive, it is almost certain that you have celiac disease. And if negative, it is almost certain that you don't. Some doctors think that a positive result warrants further gut biopsy confirmation, but others consider this test to be just as good as a gut biopsy, and perhaps better, hence avoiding further intervention. This test is also available as an inexpensive home-test kit, giving immediate results.

The symptoms of celiac disease

Another medical myth about celiac disease is that a doctor should be able to diagnose a rarely seen celiac sufferer easily from his or her symptoms. The signs, mostly emanating from the abdomen, are unmistakable, so doctors are told: chronic diarrhoea/episodic diarrhoea with malnutrition, abdominal cramping, abdominal distension or bloating, foul-smelling, bulky stools (steatorrhoea), weight loss or poor weight gain, and short stature; they should expect to also hear complaints of weakness, fatigue and loss of appetite.

Today, however, it is known that most people with celiac disease no longer go to the doctor with abdominal symptoms. Instead, patients are presenting with seemingly unrelated symptoms, such as:

- Abnormal elevation of liver enzymes of unknown cause
- Chronic nerve disease of unknown cause (such as ataxia or peripheral neuropathy)
- Chronic psychological depression
- Insulin-dependent diabetes
- Intestinal cancers
- Osteoporosis in women that is not responding to conventional therapies
- Overweight or obesity
- Permanent teeth with distinctive horizontal grooves and chalky whiteness
- Thyroid disease (both overactive and underactive)[47]

In addition, there is an increased risk of dementia and schizophrenia among patients found to have celiac disease.[48]

The osteoporosis connection

Undetected gluten sensitivity, whether or not it has led to celiac disease, is commonly found among pre- and post-menopausal women, and even children, who suffer from osteoporosis. The same nutrient deficiencies found in osteoporosis – magnesium, and vitamins D and K – are also seen in people suffering from celiac disease. In fact, one study showed that a gluten-free diet actually reversed osteoporosis in people with celiac disease.[49] The researchers took 44 celiac patients, who were aged from two to 20 years old at the time of the diagnosis, and compared them to 177 healthy, celiac-free people. The lumbar spine and whole-body bone mineral density values of people with celiac disease were significantly lower than those without. After one and a half years on a gluten-free diet, they retested the celiac group and found that their bone density had improved such that it was almost indistinguishable from that of the non-celiac sufferers.

Celiac disease and an increasing risk of cancer

Undetected celiac disease is associated with a 40–100-fold increased risk of intestinal lymphomas.[50] This is because the immune system of a person with celiac disease doesn't fight against cancer cells as well as it should. More than 80 international studies have been published on the increased incidence of cancer in celiac sufferers. In the case of intestinal lymphomas – which are the most common kind of cancer associated with celiac disease – once these are diagnosed, the prognosis is generally very poor. On the other hand, if celiac disease is diagnosed before the cancer becomes clinically evident, and a gluten-free diet is strictly followed, the risk of intestinal lymphoma decreases to near normal in five years.

The prevention of cancer is the single most compelling argument for routine and repeated screening or monitoring for celiac disease in people with any of the above conditions or symptoms or who have a close relative with celiac disease.

Can celiac sufferers eat oats?

There is growing evidence that most celiac sufferers do not react to all gluten-containing grains, but may be specifically reacting to gliadin, which is not found in oats. Oats originate from a different sub-tribe of grain to that of wheat, rye and barley, and they don't contain the same proteins. The trouble is that many oat products are contaminated with wheat, rye or barley during processing (such as milling), making them unsuitable for a gluten- or gliadin-free diet. One study found that 79 per cent of 108 oat foods analysed were severely contaminated with wheat, rye or barley, or mixtures of these three cereals.[51] The food producer, Nairn's, provides a number of guaranteed uncontaminated oat products. As to oats' safety for celiac sufferers, this is what Celiac UK says:

> Several studies have reported the safety of consuming large amounts of pure oats in people with newly diagnosed celiac

disease using clinical, serological and histological param-
eters. Research suggests that pure, uncontaminated oats
and oat products are not toxic to the majority of adults and
children with celiac disease.[52] Although it is possible that a
very small number of people with celiac disease may still be
sensitive to pure, uncontaminated oat products[53] the weight
of evidence supports the safety of oats obtained from gluten-
free manufacturers.

The cure

To date, the only known effective therapy for celiac sufferers
calls for the complete, life-long elimination of gluten/gliadin
from the diet. No wheat, rye or barley in any form is allowed
in the diet for the rest of one's life. Initially, I also recommend
the avoidance of oats; however, if an IgG food allergy test
does not show the presence of oat antibodies, then try rein-
troducing oats and monitor your symptoms. As mentioned
earlier, about 80 per cent of celiac sufferers can tolerate oats.

If a gluten-free diet is strictly followed, a dramatic resur-
gence of health should occur: diseased intestines heal,
deficient nutrients are again absorbed, bones get stronger,
and the high risk of intestinal cancer returns to a normal risk
within five years. Obviously, you first have to suspect and
diagnose celiac disease.

Healing the digestive tract

Regardless of whether or not you have celiac disease, your
'inner skin' – that is, the intestinal wall of your digestive
tract – works hard to digest and deal with the mountains of

food you eat and, as a consequence, can easily become damaged. Alcohol, antibiotics, caffeinated drinks, fried foods and
painkillers, as well as food allergens, are the most common
culprits. Painkillers can cause ulceration of the gut as I mentioned in Chapter 8. Scientists at the John Radcliffe Hospital
in Oxford who investigated NSAID side effects claim that
2,000 people in the UK die annually as a consequence of gut
damage caused by painkillers,[54] and the average person in
Britain takes over 300 painkillers a year! The result is that
the digestive tract becomes more permeable, and undigested
food proteins, instead of proteins that have broken down into
amino acids, get through the gut wall and into the bloodstream. The immune system then attacks these unwelcome
visitors. As I have explained in detail earlier, that's the basis
of most food allergies.

Glutamine – your gut's best friend

There are eight essential amino acids that your body uses
to make the protein that it requires for building and repairing. Glutamine is not one of them. Yet, despite this, it is
literally the most abundant amino acid in the human body.
There's lots of it in breast milk – five times more than any
other amino acid – and hefty amounts can be found in food;
for example, there's about 175mg of glutamine in a large
tomato, compared to less than 10mg of most other amino
acids. Why, then, does your body need all this glutamine,
and what does it do with it? It's essential for your digestive
tract, but it's also highly beneficial for your immune system
and brain.

Although most of your body's organs are fuelled by glucose,
your digestive tract is a different story. As we have seen, it's

a vast and highly active interface between your body and the outside world. It needs a lot of fuel to work properly day in and day out, and it runs on glutamine – thus sparing vital energy-giving glucose for your brain, heart and the rest of your body.

Not only does glutamine power your gut, but it heals it as well. The endothelial cells that make up the inner lining of your digestive tract replace themselves every four days and are your most critical line of defence against developing food allergies or getting infections. As your 'inner skin', your gut takes lots of hits. In Japan, it's a common practice to give patients taking non-steroidal anti-inflammatory drugs (NSAIDs) for pain and inflammation 2,000mg of glutamine 30 minutes beforehand to prevent stomach bleeding and ulceration. Many surgeons around the world now give patients glutamine after operations. The main reason is because it heals the gut and your immune system thrives off it, including vital immune cells such as lymphocytes and macrophages – they function better when they get an optimal intake of glutamine.

If you have been diagnosed with celiac disease, I recommend that you take glutamine for at least one month, ideally together with digestive enzymes and a probiotic supplement. Some supplements provide all three in one, but these don't provide enough glutamine for rapid healing. For concentrated repair during the first month, take 4–8g of glutamine a day, the equivalent of one to two heaped teaspoons of glutamine powder. (Capsules usually contain 500mg, so you'd have to take 8–16!) This will provide your gut with all the glutamine it needs to heal and rejuvenate. It's best taken last thing at night or first thing in the morning, when your stomach is empty, in a glass of water. Heat destroys glutamine, so don't take it in a hot drink. Do this every day for a month.

Beneficial bacteria – getting the balance right

Inside your body are more bacteria than living cells. Healthy bacteria flourish in a healthy digestive tract and die off in an unhealthy one. Once you've improved your digestion, re-inoculating your digestive tract with probiotics makes a big difference. These are called 'human strain' acidophilus and bifidus bacteria and work much better than dairy-derived strains found in normal yoghurt. If you do eat yoghurt, it's best to choose brands that culture their yoghurt with the acidophilus and bifidus strains of bacteria.

These friendly bacteria are not only good for your digestive tract but also for your immune system and overall health. Once you've got the correct bacterial balance in your gut, feeding the bacteria the right food helps to maintain your gut's perfect bacterial balance. What our two main beneficial bacterial species – *Lactobacillus acidophilus* and bifidobacteria – need us to eat is a diet rich in the fibre found only in fresh, unprocessed fruit, vegetables and whole, unadulterated grains. These contain a type of fibre known as prebiotics, the best known and most widely tested of which are called oligosaccharides. They also come in a supplement form, often shortened to FOS – fructo-oligosaccharides. Foods rich in prebiotics include chicory, Jerusalem artichokes and soya beans (see also page 57).

Another desirable fibre is resistant starch (see page 57), which, unlike normal starch, passes through the stomach and can only be broken down in the gut. Other favourite bacterial foods include flavonoids and lignans, found in vegetables, pulses and seeds.

If you want to give your beneficial bacteria a boost, you

might like to take a probiotic that also contains some FOS. That way you are giving the population a boost along with an added food supply. Some probiotics also contain digestive enzymes and glutamine, covering three bases in one. Taking a capsule or powder for up to 30 days is all you need to get your inner flora flourishing.

Summary – Chapter 20

My 30-day action plan for healthy celiac management is:

- Strictly avoid all wheat, rye, barley and gluten/ gliadin-containing foods. Eat only uncontaminated oats.
- Take a heaped teaspoon of glutamine powder last thing at night to improve the integrity of your digestive tract.
- Take digestive enzymes with each main meal.
- Re-inoculate your gut with beneficial bacteria by taking a capsule or powder of human-strain acidophilus and bifidobacteria. You can buy combined digestive enzymes and probiotics.
- Eat lots of vegetables, fruit and fish, and less deep-fried food, alcohol, coffee and sugar. Start each main meal with some salad or something raw.
- Chew your food well and don't eat when you're stressed.

CHAPTER 21

Ufos of the Intestines – Resolving Gut Infections

I f you are experiencing diarrhoea and abdominal pain, your body might have been invaded by a UFO – an unfriendly faecal organism. As strange as it might sound, the presence of undesirable organisms (be they bacteria, viruses or parasites) in the digestive tract is surprisingly common. In underdeveloped countries up to 99 per cent of people have been found to house parasites, according to some surveys.[55] Diarrhoea-related diseases are some of the greatest worldwide causes of mortality. Although rarely life-threatening in affluent nations, such intestinal infections are probably present in one out of four people.

A recent UK survey estimates that nine million people a year experience some kind of stomach bug, and only one in every 136 infections is reported;[56] however, many more people suffer insidious digestive symptoms that are rarely investigated. The frequency of worldwide travel is certainly one factor that has exposed more people to undesirable organisms. Many common parasites can also be encountered in water and improperly prepared food, or through poor hygiene practices and exposure to pets.

Are UFOs your problem?

Whereas diarrhoea and abdominal pain are the two most common symptoms,[57] there are many other symptoms that might lead you to suspect that you have an intestinal infection. Consider the following ten questions:

1. Do you have chronic digestive symptoms?
2. Can you trace their origin to a trip abroad, swimming in a lake, a meal or any other event that might have inadvertently exposed you to an infection?
3. Is your abdomen distended no matter what you eat?
4. Do you almost always have dark circles under your eyes?
5. Do you get diarrhoea and irregular bowel motions?
6. Do you often experience abdominal pain?
7. Do your stools frequently smell foul?
8. Do you suffer a lot from flatulence?
9. Are you finding it difficult to maintain your weight?
10. Do you often feel worse after a meal?

If you answer 'yes' to the majority of these questions, it might well be worth investigating this area further. Fortunately, parasitology tests are not only becoming more precise but also more widely available and more frequently recommended by doctors. Having said that, I have found a great deal of disparity between laboratories, based on my own personal experience. Being a keen traveller, I spent a month in Tibet and the following year made two brief trips to Turkey and Morocco. After the initial trip to Tibet, my digestion didn't seem to be as good as it used to be. I felt tired after meals, had discoloration under my eyes and experienced slight nausea. I decided to find out if I had picked up any UFOs and also to 'test the tests' at the same time. I sent off stool samples to two leading laboratories in the UK (see Resources), as well as going to see my doctor. She referred me to a specialist, who again ran a stool test for parasites. This showed nothing, while the former two laboratories both found high levels of two parasites. This is not uncommon, since some NHS laboratories do not employ the latest techniques for identifying the presence of parasites. In 1976 a Newcastle study published in the *Lancet* showed that an adult with *Giardia lamblia* needed an average of 16 consecutive investigations before their parasitic infection was diagnosed.[58] One of my favourite lab tests is the MALDI-TOF test offered by Doctor's Data (see Resources). It identifies microorganisms in a stool sample by their 'fingerprint' measured in their ribosomal protein structure. Your healthcare practitioner can arrange this kind of test.

Common parasites

The two parasites discovered in me were *Blastocystis hominis* and *Dientamoeba fragilis*. Although there are literally hundreds of possible parasites, these are two of the top ten found by parasitology laboratories. Parascope Laboratory in Leeds finds that some 40 per cent of specimens contain parasites. Genovan Diagnostics, one of the leading labs in this field, finds parasites in 20 per cent of samples tested. The Centers for Disease Control (CDC) in Atlanta, Georgia, found that one in six randomly selected people had one or more parasites. Dr Hermann Bueno is one of the world's most experienced parasitologists, and he believes that 'Parasites are the missing diagnosis in the genesis of many chronic health problems, including diseases of the gastrointestinal tract and endocrine system.'[59]

According to Antony Haynes, a clinical nutritionist specialising in the treatment of gut infections at The Nutrition Clinic in London, the following parasites are the most commonly identified in the UK:

Blastocystis hominis This is now widely considered to be a pathogen (a disease-causing organism); however, it is found in many people who have no symptoms, and should thus be treated only when symptoms are present. It can cause acute gastrointestinal (GI) symptoms when present in large numbers or in weakened individuals, as well as irritable bowel, chronic fatigue, and arthritic and rheumatic complaints. One study in Turkey found that 67 per cent of IBS sufferers were infected with *Blastocystis*.[60] It has been found in the synovial fluid in the knee of an arthritis patient. It lodges within the intestinal lining, making eradication difficult. Transmission is via contaminated food, water and surfaces; surgery; and tube-feeding in hospital.

Dientamoeba fragilis infection can be asymptomatic, or present with diarrhoea and abdominal tenderness. There may be blood in the stool. Transmission is via contaminated water or swallowing pinworm eggs in food.

Entamoeba coli infection is often asymptomatic, but might be present with mild diarrhoea. The effects of this parasite infection go beyond digestive symptoms. Their presence can lead to the development of chronic symptoms all over the body. Transmission is via cysts from water or food.

Giardia lamblia These parasites stick to the upper part of the small intestine by means of a sucking disc, coating the lining of the intestine and preventing the digestion and assimilation of food. A range of symptoms might be seen, including diarrhoea, constipation, malabsorption, fatigue, depression, bloating, flatulence, abdominal cramping, nausea and greasy stools. Whole towns and cities have been infected in recent history via contamination of the water supply (for example, Aspen, Colorado, and St Petersburg, Russia). According to the Food Standards Agency, it affects 52,000 people in the UK every year[61] and yet it is not easy to get a correct diagnosis. Transmission is via swallowing of cyst forms, which can be transported through the body, safe from destruction by digestive juices. It is at this stage that this parasite is infective because it might be transmitted by tap water or food infected with the cysts – via human or animal faeces – to another human.

Endolimax nana This is the smallest of a number of intestinal amoebas, and the most convincing research of its under-estimated virulence comes from the British researcher Dr Roger Wynburn-Mason. He suggests that *E. nana* is the cause of rheumatoid arthritis and a whole host of collagen-related diseases.[62] Some researchers believe that Wynburn-Mason might have misidentified the amoeba-like organism, although they agree that there is some kind of organism to which many individuals have become genetically susceptible, which causes rheumatoid arthritis. Transmission is via tap water or contaminated foods.

Cryptosporidium Usually the infection is short-lived in healthy people, causing abdominal discomfort, weight loss, fever, diarrhoea and nausea. In those with weak immunity, however, this parasite might result in much more severe problems because it can cause severe dehydration and electrolyte imbalances. Transmission is via contaminated ground water, farm animals, sexual contact and the faecal–oral route.

It is important to note, however, that the presence of some of these parasites doesn't necessarily mean a person will be unwell, or that they need treating. *Blastocystis hominis*, for example, is not always considered a pathogen, although there is increasing evidence that it can cause digestive problems in some people, according to Dr Ziertt at the US National Institutes of Health.[63] One of America's medical experts in the treatment of parasites, he generally only recommends treatment if there is a positive test result and associated symptoms, and especially if there is evidence of intestinal permeability (see Chapter 15). Due to the complexity of this area, if you suspect you have a problem, it is important to consult a well-informed doctor or clinical nutritionist.

Treating parasites and other UFOs

Conventional treatment of parasites, and indeed other UFOs – such as undesirable bacteria (including *Helicobacter pylori*, see Chapter 18) and yeasts (see Chapter 24) – involves a variety of antibiotic-type drugs with varying degrees of toxicity, capable of having damaging effects on beneficial intestinal bacteria. One antibiotic often prescribed in these situations is metranidazole. It is often the best choice and has a less damaging effect on healthy microbiota than other commonly used broad-spectrum antibiotics.[64] While these drug treatments might be necessary, especially for the most stubborn infections, they are often more effective if carried out alongside, or followed by, supplementation with less toxic natural remedies and probiotics using combinations of those below.

Natural remedies and their qualities

Natural Remedy	Anti-bacterial	Anti-fungal	Anti-parasitic
Berberine (an extract from goldenseal)	✔	✔	✔
Goldenseal	✔	✔	✔
Black walnut hull	✔	✔	✔
Oregano oil	✔	✔	✔
Grapefruit seed extract (citricidal)	✔	✔	✔
Garlic	✔		
Olive leaf extract	✔		
Pau d'arco		✔	
Chinese wormwood (*Artemisia annua*)	✔	✔	✔
Aloe vera	✔	✔	

There are extracts of these herbs that are more powerful than the whole herb: artemisenin, for example, the active ingredient in wormwood, can be taken in a concentrated form, which is considerably more powerful against not only a wide variety of UFOs but also against cancer cells. In oregano oil the active compound is ADP, which has a patent for its use against *Blastocystis hominis*. Oregano oil has been shown to be a particularly powerful anti-microbial agent and is a good first-line remedy to choose.[65] Some infections can be swiftly treated with natural remedies without recourse to more toxic drugs. Your health practitioner can advise you on the best strategy;

however, they are is likely to employ one or more of the above remedies. I also recommend supplementing *Saccharomyces boulardii*, which stimulates the body's own SIgA, which in turn fights off invading organisms. This is especially important if tests have shown that your SIgA level is low.

How to deal with stomach bugs

If you've been diagnosed with bacterial gastroenteritis as a result of acute symptoms of abdominal pain, diarrhoea and vomiting, you'll be prescribed antibiotics. These, however, can often make diarrhoea worse. Taking probiotics – beneficial bacteria – during an infection has been shown to halve the recovery time from diarrhoea and is therefore a wise action to take. Also, if you have been on a course of antibiotics, these disturb the normal gut bacteria that keep you healthy, and therefore you will greatly accelerate recovery to normal, healthy gut bacteria by supplementing probiotics for a few weeks after an infection.

As we have seen, the two main strains of bacteria that are resident in the human gut are *L. acidophilus* and *L. bifidus*. There is also another strain called *L. rhamnosus* (sometimes called *Lactobacillus* GG) as well as *Saccharomyces boulardii* – a type of yeast – both of which have been shown to speed up recovery from diarrhoea. (See Chapter 7 for more on this.)

L. acidophilus and *L. bifidus* are the better strains for recovery of healthy gut bacteria after taking antibiotics. A good yoghurt is one source, but you must make sure it has been cultured with *Lactobacillus acidophilus* and bifidobacteria, which most are not. A guaranteed alternative is supplementation. These are best taken on an empty stomach. Also, take them away from antibiotics.

High-dose vitamin C helps

Vitamin C is both antibacterial and antiviral, but it is most effective against viruses. Many cases of gastroenteritis are caused by viruses such as the rotavirus and norovirus. High-dose vitamin C can help to speed up recovery, but it is a double-edged sword, because too much can induce diarrhoea. The optimal dose is the amount just below that which causes loose bowels (this is called 'bowel tolerance').

Vitamin C is flushed out of the body in a few hours, and so the best results are achieved by taking 500–1,000mg every one or two hours during infection. Pure vitamin C is ascorbic acid. A gentler, alkaline form is called ascorbate. Since dehydration is the major problem to watch out for (see below), mixing sodium ascorbate powder with water and a little juice, and sipping that mixture regularly, is a good way to take high-dose vitamin C. Vitamin C also helps antibiotics to work.

High-dose B_3 (niacinamide) kills superbugs

Superbugs, such as antibiotic-resistant staph infections, are becoming a real problem, killing thousands of people worldwide. Researchers from the Linus Pauling Institute have found that high-dose vitamin B_3 increased by 1,000 times the ability of immune cells to kill staph bacteria.[66] The work was done both in laboratory animals and with human blood. The vitamin, given in the form of niacinamide, dramatically boosted natural immunity, increasing the numbers and efficacy of neutrophils, a specialised type of white blood cell that can kill and consume harmful bacteria. In human blood, clinical doses of vitamin B_3 appeared to wipe out the staph infection in only a few hours. Although human trials are yet to be done, it suggests that high-dose niacinamide – that is, 1,000–3,000mg of niacinamide – could make a big difference to fighting bacterial infections. It is not harmful, especially for short-term use. The RDA (recommended daily allowance) for vitamin B_3 is 18mg, so this is way beyond any amount that could be achieved through diet.

Garlic and grapefruit seed extract

Garlic contains allicin, which is anti-viral, anti-fungal and anti-bacterial. Rich in sulphur-containing amino acids, it also acts as an antioxidant. It is undoubtedly an important ally in fighting infections. Consider taking one garlic clove daily, for example, if you are travelling in regions where food poisoning is more common.

Grapefruit seed extract is an anti-microbial agent. The great advantage, however, is that it doesn't adversely affect beneficial gut bacteria. It is available in drops, is antiseptic, and can be swallowed, gargled, or used as nose or ear drops, depending on the site of infection. This is a good all-rounder to have if you are travelling. You need about 20 drops two or three times a day if you have an infection, or ten drops, or a capsule a day, as a preventative. In my experience, it is less potent that *Artemisia annua*: I usually travel with a concentrated tincture of this, which is also a well-tolerated anti-malarial, taking ten drops twice a day.

Keep well hydrated

The major danger from gastroenteritis is becoming chronically dehydrated. If you have acute diarrhoea, dry mouth, sunken eyes and are feeling extremely weak and not peeing much at all, it is vital to see a doctor and get some hydration salts, which are added to water. If the body loses too much liquid through acute diarrhoea, vital minerals, including sodium (salt) get depleted. For this reason it is important to keep drinking. You can buy rehydration salts in any pharmacist, to add to water.

Although you might not feel like eating, the immune system needs protein to stay strong. Eating soups made with beans, lentils or meat stock is a gentle way to keep nourished and hydrated.

How to prevent infections

Prevention is better than cure, and the best way to stay free of UFOs and gut infections is to ensure that your immune system is fighting fit, your intestinal flora is flourishing, your digestive system is healthy and your exposure to potential UFOs is minimised.

The most common foods to cause food poisoning are undercooked meat and chicken, unfresh fish and shellfish – especially tuna – eggs, and also leafy greens that have been exposed to contaminated animal manure or contaminated water.

The following habits can help to reduce your risk:

- Drink filtered, distilled, bottled or boiled water, especially when abroad.
- Wash fruit and vegetables thoroughly. Eat fresh food, ideally grown locally and organically.
- Wash your hands with soap before eating, and keep your fingernails short and clean.

- Cook food at the correct temperature (above 100°C) to kill parasites and bacteria. Cook meat at 170°C or above, and bake fish at 200°C. Many incidences result from eating at restaurants with unhygienic practices, such as thawing and refreezing food.
- Avoid raw foods, such as sushi, as well as shellfish and crab unless you know it is fresh and of good quality.
- Eat only free-range fresh eggs, discarding those with broken shells, and cooking well.
- Sanitise all toilet seats and bowls, especially those used by children.
- Be careful about walking barefoot, especially in warm, moist, sandy soil.
- Don't use tap water to clean contact lenses. Use sterilised lens solutions.
- Keep toddlers away from puppies and kittens that have not been regularly wormed, and don't let them kiss animals.

Supplementary benefit

I recommend these supplements to help you get back on your feet:

2 × high-potency multivitamin and mineral with at least 10mg of zinc

4–10 × vitamin C 1,000mg, ideally with zinc up to bowel tolerance, or the equivalent of 10g a day of sodium ascorbate dissolved in water, or more, up to bowel tolerance

2 × *Lactobacillus acidophilus* and bifidobacteria, giving 5–10 billion active organisms, ideally away from food or before meals

1–2 teaspoons (5–10g) glutamine powder in water, last thing at night on an empty stomach

Optional (for bacterial infections, especially staph)

2–3 × niacinamide (B$_3$) 500mg (not niacin – a form of B$_3$ that makes you blush when taken in high doses)

CAUTIONS: If you are not better within a few days, or your symptoms are acute, or if you have any signs of dehydration, it is very important to seek immediate medical attention.

Don't take iron supplements, or a multivitamin that contains iron, at the same time as antibiotics, as iron reduces the absorption of some antibiotics.

Summary – Chapter 21

In summary, if you do have a persistent gut infection, or symptoms that suggest this:

- It is vital to get properly diagnosed. You may need referral to a gastroenterologist for this.
- Also see a nutritional therapist, who can arrange a gut parasitology test.
- Boost your gut's defences with daily probiotics.
- If you know the kind of infection you have, you can use the remedies indicated above but do seek medical advice if your symptoms persist.
- Follow the guidelines above for preventing infections if you are travelling in high-risk areas.

CHAPTER 22

How to Prevent Bloating, Wind and Water Retention

Two-thirds of people report suffering from bloating. In the Holford 100% Health Survey of over 55,000 people, 65 per cent reported frequently or occasionally experiencing bloating, and 59 per cent reported flatulence. There are two main causes of bloating: one is gas and the other is water.

I remember my first client who, on eliminating their food intolerances, lost 3.2kg/7lb in two days. Now, I thought, that cannot be fat loss. To lose 1kg/2lb of fat in a week is good going. You have to be cutting down calories, eating a low-GL diet and exercising. More than two-thirds of your body is made up of water, and the body can sometimes retain too much, creating unnecessary weight gain. This can be a consequence of poor kidney function, hormonal imbalances and too much sugar. The body stores excess sugar as glycogen, each unit of which is bound to four units of water. In addition, one very common cause of waterlogging is food intolerance. Ask yourself the following questions:

1. Does your face look puffy, especially around the eyes?
2. Does your abdomen, on pressing, feel bloated?
3. Do your arms or thighs feel puffy rather than being pure fat and muscle?
4. Do your ankles ever swell up?
5. Do your fingers ever swell up so that it's hard to get your rings off?
6. Do you have dry skin or dandruff?
7. Do you ever experience sudden fluctuations in your weight?
8. Do you suffer from breast tenderness?
9. Are you prone to allergies or intolerances?

If you answered yes to three or more of the questions above, the chances are that water retention is partly to blame for your weight problem.

The role of food intolerances and water retention

As I have explained earlier, if an unwanted substance (such as an indigested protein) passes across the wall of your digestive tract and into the bloodstream, your immune system reacts. But why does it lead to water retention and weight gain? The reason is twofold. First, histamine release, which is what makes you sneeze if you have hay fever, makes tiny blood vessels, called capillaries, more leaky. This allows the immune system's army of white blood cells to move into the battlefield. At the same time, more fluid passes into your tissues. If this is happening several times a day, you become waterlogged. Immune reactions also mess up the balance of prostaglandins – the hormone-like substances made from essential fats – and this too can lead to water retention, as well as abdominal bloating. Food intolerances and allergies cause the release of histamine and other inflammatory molecules.

This is not the only mechanism that might link food intolerances to weight gain. When your immune system is frequently reacting to the foods you eat, you develop a background of chronic inflammation and that, in turn, can impair the brain's ability to receive the appetite-suppressant leptin's messages (this is called leptin resistance),[67] so you keep eating. Removing foods from the diet that are provoking the inflammation can help undo the damage, reducing weight and moderating appetite.

That's the theory, but where is the proof? YorkTest, Britain's most advanced and science-led food intolerance laboratory, recently surveyed 38 individuals who had taken a food-specific IgG test and who had reported weight loss after making dietary changes according to the test results. According to Dr Gill Hart, the scientific director, however: 'Only 13 per cent stated that weight loss was the primary reason for using the programme. Other primary reasons for using the programme included digestive symptoms such as IBS and bloating (47 per cent), skin symptoms such as eczema and rashes (11 per cent), migraines (2.5 per cent), fatigue (2.5 per cent), and other (24 per cent). Half said that they were concerned about their weight before they took the test. One in four (26 per cent) noticed a reduction in weight within a week. A further 26 per cent said they lost weight between 1 and 2 weeks, 31 per cent between 2 and 4 weeks, and 17 per cent took more than 4 weeks. The majority (92 per cent) said that the weight loss that they achieved was desirable. Fourteen per cent lost up to 5lb, 34 per cent lost between 6 and 10lb, 26 per cent lost between 11 and 15lb, 17 per cent lost between 16 and 20lb and 9 per cent lost over 20lb in weight over a greater than 3 month period by avoiding their intolerant foods, identified by YorkTest's Food and Drink Scan Programme. Not only that, their weight loss was sustained and often manageable for the first time.'

The most common kind of immune reaction to foods isn't a food allergy (an IgE-mediated immune response) but a food intolerance, which leads to the production of IgG antibodies. These induce an IgG immune reaction when the trigger foods are eaten. As we have seen, the symptoms can often be a delayed reaction, making it difficult to identify the offending foods. They also cause fluid retention.

The YorkTest findings are completely consistent with a previously published study in the US, which reported an average 5.4kg/12lb weight loss after 60 days in a group of 120 people tested for and avoiding their IgG-positive foods using Immuno Laboratory's test.[68] They also had desirable reductions in waist and hip circumferences, blood pressure and quality-of-life indicators.

The more foods you eat that provoke an IgG antibody reaction, the worse it is for your health and your weight. Your immune system is not designed to produce large amounts of IgG antibodies. If it does, you are likely to suffer from some degree of discomfort and symptoms that just don't seem to improve, as well as being resistant to weight loss. If you suspect that you may have reactions to foods, I recommend that you investigate further by having a IgG food intolerance test, which you can do with a simple home test kit (see Resources). The results are sent to you, showing you exactly which foods your immune system is reacting against. Also, unlike the classic IgE-mediated food allergy, IgG sensitivities don't always last for life. These sensitivities often disappear after a few months if you stop eating your offending foods and at the same time improve your diet and take supplements con-taining digestive enzymes, glutamine and probiotics to keep your gut healthy.

Case Study: Cathy

Cathy took a food intolerance test after suffering with prolonged digestive problems. The constipation, wind and bloating she was experiencing were all classic symptoms of irritable bowel syndrome (IBS). So severe was her condition that she frequently had to visit the hospital. The tests she underwent could not identify the root cause of the problem, and the medication she was prescribed only made her feel worse. Not only were her symptoms uncomfortable and at times pain-ful, but they also caused her great embarrassment.

> 'When I say I was "bloated" it doesn't really do justice to my symptoms. I was carrying so much fluid that I felt constantly swollen. I was asked on a regular basis if I was pregnant and when was I due. It was terribly upsetting and humiliating, and to add to the problem my weight started going up even though I had never had a problem with my weight in the past. I felt very down and depressed, and I suffered with low esteem, so for two years I didn't go out and couldn't socialise. I hated looking in the mirror, and I had a very poor image of myself.'

After struggling with the combination of her weight gain, poor health and the negative impact on her mood, Cathy decided to try a different route to get to the cause of her problems.

'One day my mum suggested that I take a food intolerance test to see if that could help with my symptoms. I decided to give it a go as I hadn't had any luck through doctors and the hospital.'

When she received her results, Cathy learnt she was reacting to egg white, egg yolk and, surprisingly, peas. To better understand the changes she needed to make to her diet and to ensure that she replaced her trigger foods with nutritious alternatives, she booked a consultation with a nutritional therapist, who talked her through the results and helped her to plan delicious, satisfying meals.

'I immediately took eggs out of my diet and replaced them with porridge for breakfast, and the effect was almost immediate. I instantly felt like I had more energy, and after a couple of weeks my swollen stomach went flat for the first time in years!'

Now, armed with the knowledge of her food intolerance and supported by the advice of her nutritional therapist, Cathy has been able to manage her health and weight and is looking forward to a bright future.

'With my new increased energy levels I am able to go to the gym more, and my weight has come down from 10 stone 2 pounds to 7 stone 11 pounds in 7 months. My depression has totally lifted and my whole attitude to food and life has changed. I am delighted to see my body changing and my new shape. My confidence levels have soared and I couldn't be happier.'

The causes of wind

The digestive tract usually contains about 200ml of gas, and it is not abnormal to pass 400–2,000ml of this daily. About 90 per cent of the gas is made up of nitrogen, oxygen, carbon dioxide, methane and hydrogen. The nitrogen and oxygen come from air that is swallowed; the carbon dioxide is produced when stomach acid mixes with bicarbonates in bile and pancreatic juices. Most of the oxygen and carbon dioxide are reabsorbed into the bloodstream through the small intestine. As we have seen, the colon, or large bowel, contains billions of bacteria, which are essential for good health and whose job it is to ferment products that pass from the small intestine. As the bacteria ferment, the residues, large amounts of hydrogen, methane, carbon dioxide and other gases are produced. Although some of these are reabsorbed into the blood and excreted in the breath, the rest is passed as wind.

One of the major causes of excessive wind is dysbiosis and indigestion (see Chapters 14 and 17). If food is not completely broken down, this provides microorganisms in the digestive tract with more 'food' – hence more gas. The first step to solving this problem is to change your diet and to supplement digestive enzymes with each meal (see Chapter 2). Certain foods do generate more gas, including beans and some vegetables such as cabbage, Brussels sprouts, cauliflower, turnips, leeks, onions and garlic.

Poor digestion and dysbiosis

Although food intolerance is a common cause of bloating, some people just aren't good at digesting certain foods and they consequently bloat. The effect can be almost immediate, within less than an hour of eating the food. The logical explanation is that if the digestive system doesn't digest the food adequately, the bacteria in the guts will feed on it, producing gas and hence bloating. This may or may not be the true and only explanation for sudden bloating, but I have had many patients who have experienced almost immediate relief from taking digestive enzymes. It might be that their body is already 'primed' by virtue of having a degree of dysbiosis and an unhealthy balance of bacteria waiting to pounce on undigested food. An overgrowth of bacteria in the small intestine is a likely candidate for contributing to bloating, as in an overgrowth of the *Candida albicans* yeast (see Chapter 24). I discuss this as a cause of irritable bowel syndrome in the next chapter.

The most common offending foods for wind are beans, lentils and other pulses, which require alpha-galactosidase for their digestion; and greens, especially cruciferous vegetables (cabbage, Brussels sprouts, cauliflower), which require amyloglucosidase (also called glucoamylase). Certain others generate more gas, including turnips, leeks, onions and garlic. Beans, onions and garlic are also high in resistant starch. Some people who have difficulties with these foods do well on a low-FODMAP diet (see page 241), which eliminates resistant starches. Other people are intolerant to the sugar in milk, lactose, and bloat unless they supplement the enzyme lactase.

If you bloat after these foods, you might also like to try taking a digestive enzyme containing alpha-galactosidase and amyloglucosidase, plus the basics for digesting protein (protease), carbohydrate (amylase) and fat (lipase). Some enzyme supplements include probiotics, which is not a bad idea in any case. Read Chapter 2 for more on digestive enzymes.

Check your hormones

Although the effect is not immediate, if you are prone to bloating and/or water retention, one possible contributor is hormone imbalance. Oestrogen dominance – relatively more oestrogen than progesterone – is extremely common in women in the peri- and menopausal years. This is due to anovulatory cycles, because progesterone is only produced if ovulation has occurred. Oestrogen is also produced in fat cells, so this is more likely in overweight women. This can trigger more water and sodium to enter the cells, thereby causing water retention and often an increase in blood pressure. If you do have a lack of progesterone, correcting this can lead to a reduction in bloating and water retention with its consequent weight loss.

Summary – Chapter 22

If you often experience bloating:

- Quit sugar and follow a low-GL diet.
- Rule out kidney problems if you have the symptoms of excessive water retention.
- Find out if you have any food intolerances, and eliminate them.
- Have a trial period taking digestive enzymes with probiotics with each main meal to find out whether you are struggling to digest certain foods.

CHAPTER 23

Solving the Riddle of Irritable Bowel Syndrome

I rritable bowel syndrome (IBS) is not one disease with a single cause, but a broad term used to describe several, sometimes contradictory symptoms. The effects can be random and can disappear as spontaneously as they come on, although for many people it is a chronic condition. All this apparent vagueness does not make for an easy diagnosis or treatment but, with such a high incidence, this problem – also known as intestinal neurosis, spastic colitis, spastic colon or mucous colitis – demands a solution. Many sufferers find anti-spasmodic drugs, fibre supplements and laxatives prescribed by their doctors unhelpful. In the absence of any proven cause, quite a few people are offered antidepressants on the basis that it must be 'in the mind'. IBS is the second highest cause of absenteeism after the common cold, with 20 per cent of the adult population experiencing bouts of it. Twice as many women as men are said to suffer from it, although this might just be because women are more likely to report the symptoms.

If you have any or all of the following symptoms,

continually or recurrently for at least three months, there is a strong possibility that you have IBS:

abdominal pain
anxiety
bloating
constipation
cramps
depression
diarrhoea
gas
mucus in stools
nausea

Whatever the cause of the symptoms that can be described as IBS, the common thread is a disturbance to the usual control of the bowel by a complex set of nerves, which determines its movements and the substances it secretes. Normally, digestion is regulated in part by the autonomic branch of the nervous system (ANS), which controls involuntary bodily functions such as the beating of the heart and the secretion of hormones. In a healthy gut, the ANS moves food along with rhythmic contractions, but in the case of IBS the muscles go into spasm. The mechanisms by which the ANS works are very subtle and therefore easily disrupted, and they are intricately linked with the gut's production of neurotrans-mitters and its other communication systems, including the GALT (gut-associated lymphatic tissue), designed to react to substances and situations that are not favourable. When this happens, food and waste material do not move along the digestive tract normally, so mucus and toxins accumulate, and gas and stools become trapped, causing bloating and pain, which often worsen with eating and are relieved by a bowel movement. Women often find their symptoms worsen around the time of their period.

IBS or inflammatory bowel disease?

One distinguishing feature of IBS – compared with other bowel complaints – is the apparent lack of changes visible in bowel tissue (in contrast to Crohn's disease where the digestive tract becomes ulcerated). This has prevented IBS from being classified as an inflammatory bowel disease. However, research at the Technische Universität München (aptly abbreviated to TUM) has discovered that mini inflammations in the gut upset the sensitive balance of the bowel.[69] The lead researcher, Professor Schemann, put it this way, 'The irritated mucosa releases increased amounts of neuroactive substances such as serotonin, histamine and protease. This cocktail could be the real cause of the unpleasant symptoms of IBS.' Why this inflammation occurs I will address shortly.

Another feature of IBS is that, despite symptoms, sufferers' overall health is good, without the serious factors such as weight loss, fever, bleeding or anaemia that occur with other bowel disorders. Before any treatment of suspected IBS, it is important to consult your GP to rule out other conditions that might be linked to similar symptoms, including diverticulitis, infectious diarrhoea, inflammatory bowel disease (for example, Crohn's or ulcerative colitis), diabetes, cancer, laxative abuse, mechanical problems, such as impacted faeces, and celiac disease.

Back in 1892, Sir William Osler wrote in *The Principles and Practice of Medicine* of mucous colitis, describing 'a tenacious mucus, which may be slimy and gelatinous, like frog-spawn' in patients who were often hysterical and depressed. IBS, then, is not entirely a modern disease, yet the alarming prevalence of IBS in developed countries is just one indication that it is a condition that is largely due to diet and lifestyle.

Because there is no test for IBS as such, it is essential to create a picture of what is causing the symptoms for each individual – be it food intolerances, dysbiosis, stress, hormone changes, dietary factors, including low fibre consumption, infection or other factors. A practitioner therefore has to take a careful history of the client's symptoms, diet and lifestyle in order to determine the cause of the IBS. Dr Jean Munro, medical director of the Brakespear Hospital for Allergy and Environmental Medicine, believes, 'It's practically always associated with food reactions as well as some form of dysbiosis.'

IBS, food allergy and intolerance

Food sensitivities in people with IBS have been recognised since the turn of the twentieth century and are found in as many as two-thirds of sufferers. In people who have allergies or who come from families with allergies, this must be a prime consideration; however, IgE antibody level, which is the basis for conventional allergies, has not been shown to be higher in IBS sufferers compared to normal, healthy people. IgG antibodies, on the other hand, which are associated with food intolerances, are often higher. Researchers at St George's Hospital Medical School in London measured both types of antibodies in 108 people with IBS, and compared the levels with 43 healthy controls. The researchers found that the people with IBS had significantly higher levels of IgG antibodies to specific foods, including wheat, beef, lamb, pork and soya. Both groups had raised IgG antibody levels to dairy products. Neither group, however, had raised levels of IgE antibodies.[70]

IgG reactions are more often associated with bloating, IBS, headaches, chronic tiredness and aching joints. Once you know the foods that your system is reacting to – wheat, milk and yeast being the most common – you can omit these foods from your diet and give your digestive system a break. The odds are quite high that you'll benefit. Researchers from Monash University in Australia, headed by Dr Jessica Biesiekierski, put non-celiac volunteers on a gluten-free diet and reported improvements in bloating, abdominal pain, stool consistency and tiredness.[71] As we have seen, there is growing recognition that many people without celiac disease do react to wheat gluten. Exactly how is a subject of much research. Many IBS sufferers also find improvement on a lactose-free diet. One study of 70 IBS sufferers found a quarter were lactose intolerant and most (87 per cent) benefited from a lactose-free diet.[72] Lactose intolerance is more common among people of Asian and African ancestry. You can also be allergic (IgE) or intolerant (IgG) to dairy protein, and not just unable to digest the milk sugar lactose; for example, I am not lactose intolerant, but I am allergic to dairy.

Knowing that IBS sufferers have significantly raised levels of IgG antibodies to specific foods, researchers at the University of York devised an ingenious study[73] to discover if cutting out these foods made a difference.

They ran an IgG test on 150 IBS sufferers and then gave their doctors either the real or fake results, along with a diet to follow for three months. Those with the fake results were given a list of random foods to avoid. At the end of the period only those following a diet based on avoiding the foods highlighted as problematic on their test results reported a significant improvement. What's more, those who stuck to it most strictly had the best results. Level of compliance, on the other hand, didn't make a difference in those on the sham diets. Compared to patients given the commonly prescribed drug Tegaserod, those following the allergy-free diet were seven times more likely to benefit.

Other clinical studies have found the most commonly offending foods to be grains (especially wheat), dairy products, coffee, tea and citrus fruits. Intolerance of lactose is particularly common, while other sugars, even those in fruits, can cause problems too.

In surveys, three out of four IBS sufferers report significant improvement from avoiding IgG-positive foods. The Olympic athlete, Denise Lewis, is an example:

Case Study: Denise

'Since removing my allergy foods a year ago, I haven't had a single IBS attack. It's not always easy to avoid the foods, but the benefits are worth it for a pain-free existence. Finding out what I'm allergic to with an IgG allergy test has transformed my life. For the first time in 13 years I'm pain free.'

Many IBS sufferers find relief by avoiding gluten (wheat, rye, barley), but it is usually those with diarrhoea who find they do better without dairy products. It is, however, important not to jump to conclusions. One patient of mine, who suffered with terrible IBS and bloating, was convinced that she was intolerant to wheat. She described an incident where she went to an Indian restaurant, ordered a curry, a naan bread and a lager and bloated so badly her trousers split. She had to make a strategic retreat from the restaurant!

When I tested her, however, she was intolerant to yeast and cashew nuts, not wheat. There was yeast in the bread and the lager, and cashews in the curry.

Food intolerances are frequently linked to leaky gut syndrome (see Chapter 15). This in itself can cause a host of problems, including depressed immunity and fatigue. If IBS is persistent, it may well be linked to leaky gut, in which case steps must be taken to heal the gut lining using dietary changes and supplements, such as zinc, vitamin A, essential fats and glutamine. Tests are available from nutritional thera-pists to determine gut permeability.

Some so-called health experts are sceptical about food intolerances, however, claiming that they are all in the mind. An example of this is a recent study from the Institute of Medicine at the University of Bergen. They found that in a group of people self-reporting food hypersensitivity 89 per cent had IBS and 57 per cent tested positive for a psychological problem, anxiety and depression being the most common.[74] They ran serum tests for IgE, and also took skin-prick tests which also involve IgE-based antibody reactions, and found no real correlation. Of course, you can interpret these results in three ways. Either you say that IBS is 'in the mind', or that there's a common underlying cause for both IBS and psychological symptoms; although, it is important to realise that other studies show no correlation between IgE antibodies and IBS but a strong correlation between IgG antibodies – the marker for food intolerance – and IBS, as we have been discussing in this chapter, and that sufferers have found significant relief when avoiding their offending foods. The third interpretation, then, is that the study's authors measured the wrong kind of marker for food intolerance.

Digestive enzymes and dysbiosis

Other problems of digestion are also linked to IBS: a lack of digestive enzymes being one of them. Some foods, such as pulses, beans, nuts and cauliflower, contain a carbohydrate that is inherently difficult to digest. A specific digestive enzyme – alpha-galactosidase – helps to break it down. Other than intolerances of specific foods, a diet that is low in nutrients, fresh foods and fibre (excluding wheat bran, which can irritate the gut) can trigger digestive and other disorders. Such a diet invariably causes constipation and an imbalance in gut flora (dysbiosis) that ultimately causes a build-up of toxic matter in the lining of the intestines; IBS is just one possible outcome.

Probiotics can also help with IBS.[75] A commercial product containing inulin, called Bimuno, was found to help IBS patients. It boosted the numbers of the beneficial bifido-bacteria and reduced the levels of several harmful bacteria, such as clostridium. Symptoms, such as pain and bloating, improved.[76] People with IBS are most often reported to have a low level of bifidobacteria. A study in Finland found that those who reported abdominal pain had five times lower levels of bifidobacteria than those who didn't have these symptoms.[77]

Altering your diet and taking supplements of beneficial bacteria (or other substances, such as butyric acid or fructo-oligosaccharides, that encourage their growth) will help to repopulate the intestinal environment with these essential friends. An overgrowth of the yeast *Candida albicans*, a relatively common problem which sometimes accompanies IBS, requires special dietary strategies (discussed in Chapter 24). The number of parasites that inhabit our intestines might be quite alarming; most produce no symptoms, but others can give rise to IBS, gastrointestinal disorders and other health problems. Most common are *Giardia lamblia* and *Blastocystis hominis* (see Chapter 21).

Small intestinal bacterial overgrowth

In his book *The Digestive Health Solution*, naturopath Benjamin Brown places a big emphasis on the overgrowth of bacteria in the small intestine, known as SIBO, as a frequent cause of IBS. This results in more fermentation and gas, present in 84 per cent of IBS sufferers, according to one study. The authors of this study then gave an antibiotic that acts locally in the gut, and is not absorbed, which resulted in a 75 per cent relief of all symptoms.[78] 'People with SIBO also tend to have higher levels of bad bacteria including *Escheriichia coli* (*E. coli*), *Enterococcus* and *Klebsiella pneumonia*,'[79] says Brown. 'Overgrowth of these bad bugs results in the production of bacterial toxins, which can activate your immune system, causing damage to the gut wall, inflammation, increased sensitivity, pain, constipation and diarrhoea.'[80]

A nutritional therapist can arrange for you to have a stool test, which will establish levels of bacteria, both good and bad, in the gut.

The possibility of SIBO is particularly relevant if the onset of IBS symptoms coincided with a gut infection, or a course of antibiotics, or the use of antacid PPI drugs. One study of people experiencing acid reflux who were given PPIs found that after eight weeks of drug treatment 48 per cent were complaining of bloating, flatulence, abdominal pain or diarrhoea – the symptoms of IBS. Six months on, 26 per cent had developed SIBO and many had developed IBS.[81]

The low-FODMAP diet

At various points in this book I've extolled the merits of slow-releasing carbohydrates, low-GI sugars and resistant starches that act as prebiotics, feeding bacteria in the gut. One problem with these prebiotics is that, if you have an overgrowth of non-beneficial bacteria in the gut, as in SIBO, these otherwise healthy foods might actually encourage growth of those bacteria.

Some IBS sufferers do particularly badly on these soluble-fibre-rich foods, developing excessive gas. For these people, a low-FODMAP diet can provide relief. What does FODMAP mean?

- The 'F' in FODMAP stands for fermentable or 'creating gas'.
- 'O' stands for oligosaccharides: water-soluble fibres that are found in wheat, garlic, onion, barley, rye, chicory root and its extract (inulin), which are added to many foods to boost their fibre content.
- 'D' stands for disaccharides, which is the lactose found in milk, yoghurt and ice cream.
- 'M' stands for monosaccharide or the sugar fructose, when it is present in foods in quantities that exceed their glucose content – found in some apples, pears, watermelon, honey and agave syrup.
- 'P' is for polyols, which are sugar alcohols found in peaches, plums, apples, cauliflower and mushrooms, and added as artificial sweeteners to sugar-free gum, mints and some medications – also the low-GL sweetener xylitol.

The theory is that these carbohydrates cause gas production, which stretches the intestinal wall and stimulates the nerves in the gut. It is this stretching that triggers the sensations of pain and discomfort that are commonly experienced by IBS sufferers. Clinical studies of IBS sufferers following the low-FODMAP diet have generally had very positive results. A recent study followed up 131 IBS sufferers and 49 inflammatory bowel disease sufferers who had been put on the low-FODMAP diet.[82] Of those who stuck to the diet there was significant relief, especially with regard to bloating and abdominal pain. Forty-two per cent of those with inflammatory bowel disease had a very positive improvement in symptoms, compared to 23 per cent of IBS sufferers. Since this diet is not easy to follow, it is particularly interesting that the food groups most often not reintroduced were dairy products, wheat products and onions. Dairy products and wheat are also the most common food allergens.

The low-FODMAP diet might be successful because (a) it inhibits growth of unfriendly bacteria in people with SIBO, and (b) it might eliminate foods that many people have intolerances to. That is, of course, a good thing, but it's a bit hit and miss. If you can afford to have a test to establish whether you have a bacterial imbalance, and then you correct it with the appropriate probiotics, and if you can discover which precise foods you are intolerant to, and eliminate them, you might find relief without having to eliminate all the FODMAP foods, many of which are positively healthy, provided you don't have SIBO or a specific food intolerance.

FODMAP foods to eat and those to avoid

Foods to eat	Foods to avoid
Meat and fish: All types	
Dairy and fats: Butter Eggs Hard cheeses (such as Parmesan) Lactose-free ice creams or desserts Nuts and nut butters (but avoid pistachio nuts) Milk substitutes, such as nut or rice milks or lactose-free milk Vegetable oils and olive oil Yoghurt (if natural and low lactose – see if you can tolerate it)	**Dairy:** Cream Cream cheese Ice cream Milk Milk products (creamer, instant milk powder, cocoa, etc.) Soft cheese Sweetened/flavoured yoghurts
Grains/cereals: Amaranth Buckwheat Corn/polenta Millet Oats Quinoa Rice Tapioca/cassava Teff	**Grains/cereals:** Barley (pearl and pot) Bulgar wheat Couscous (contains wheat) Rye Semolina (contains wheat) Wheat and wheat products (bread, pasta, cake, biscuits, etc.)

Foods to eat	Foods to avoid
Vegetables:	**Vegetables:**
Aubergine (some people can't tolerate)	Artichokes
	Asparagus
Baby corn (well-cooked)	Avocado
Carrots	Beans and pulses (legumes)
Celery	Beetroot
Courgette	Cabbage
Green beans	Cauliflower
Lettuce	Broccoli
Pak choi/choy sum	Garlic
Peppers	Mushrooms
Potatoes	Onions
Spinach	Peas
Spring onion (green part only)	Sugar snaps/mangetouts
Swede	Shallots
Yams/sweet potato	Fennel
Parsnip	
Squash	
Tomatoes	
Fruit:	**Fruit:**
Banana	Apple
Grapes	Apricot
Grapefruit	Peach
Honeydew melon	Cherries
Cantaloupe melon	Blackberries
Kiwi fruit	Mango
Lemon/lime	Dried fruit (in large quantities)
Orange	Nectarine
Pineapple	Pear
Rhubarb	Plum
Raspberries	Prune
Strawberries	Watermelon
Blueberries	
Cranberries	

If you do suffer from IBS, following a low-FODMAP diet in the short term might make a big difference. During an attack of IBS, it's best to choose low-FODMAP-friendly foods without too high a fibre content, and you can also take slippery elm tea. Charcoal tablets can be used to relieve occasional gas and bloating, but it is important to eliminate the cause, rather than just dealing with the symptoms. In the long term, if you respond to the FODMAP approach you'll need to dig deeper to find out what's going on in your gut to make your system so hypersensitive to otherwise healthy foods.

Use the following list of general dietary tips to help alleviate IBS:

- Eliminate suspected food allergens and intolerances based on IgG testing.
- Eat plenty of fresh vegetables.
- Eat simple meals and chew thoroughly.
- Increase soluble fibre (not wheat bran), especially in cases of constipation.
- Drink plenty of water, herbal teas and diluted juices.
- Avoid foods rich in sulphur, as they can cause wind (bread, eggs, onions and most dried fruits).
- Avoid sugar.
- Avoid wheat (even in people who are not sensitive it can irritate the gut).
- Avoid refined/processed foods.
- Avoid dairy products (especially in cases of diarrhoea).
- Limit or avoid alcohol, coffee, tea and cigarettes.
- Avoid spicy foods.

As we have seen, we all have numerous bacteria and other microorganisms living in our guts. Problems arise when unfriendly bacteria outnumber the friendly ones, or are toxic, or others (such as yeasts) multiply to such an extent that they disrupt digestive function. Such imbalances (discussed fully in Chapters 7 and 14) often accompany IBS. Using antibiotics and antacids can contribute to dysbiosis by disturbing the delicate balance of microflora throughout the digestive tract.

You might also benefit from increasing your intake of anti-inflammatory foods (see Chapter 19). A recent study using a herbal extract of berberine, found in goldenseal, reported substantial improvement in diarrhoea among those with IBS.[83]

Nerves, spasms – and peppermint oil

As mentioned earlier, the functioning of the digestive tract is subject to the intricate workings of the autonomic nervous system (ANS), which we do not consciously control, and any disruption to this can have far-reaching effects. Stress to the body – whether it is a strong emotion, anxiety, illness or even the presence of an allergenic food or toxin – will set alarm bells ringing. In such a situation, the ANS perceives 'danger' and diverts energy from the body's systems, such as digestion, that are not immediately required to deal with the 'emergency'. As you can imagine, shutting down the digestive system is likely to result in constipation and a build-up of toxins. In some situations, however, the ANS reaction is so strong that it results in immediate diarrhoea. The ANS might be triggered by something psychological or something physical, such as bloating, extending and stretching the gut wall. Some people do get relief from anti-spasmodic drugs, but these have known side effects.

I prefer to recommend peppermint oil as a natural anti-spasmodic. It has proven just as effective as anti-spasmodic drugs,[84] reducing muscle spasms, cramping and pain.[85] It is very well researched and also seems to kill off bad bacteria and even help SIBO.[86]

Make sure you use an enteric-coated capsule of peppermint oil to prevent it breaking down in the stomach so that it can act effectively in the small intestine. The dose that has proven effective is 0.2ml three times a day.

The stress connection

Obviously, not everyone who gets stressed (all of us do, at some time) suffers from IBS, but there is a clear link between the two. An article in the *Lancet* suggests that 'anxiety is a predisposing factor'.[87] The other side of the coin is that people suffering from a long-term, frustrating condition such as IBS are likely to become anxious or depressed, as shown in numerous studies. Regardless of which comes first – IBS or stress of any sort – many sufferers have found great relief when they combine treatment with behavioural therapies such as stress management, counselling or hypnotherapy. Herbs such as skullcap, valerian and passionflower can be useful for calming the ANS. Other practices – such as yoga, t'ai chi, regular exercise, taking time to eat, chewing well and not eating less than two hours before bedtime – also promote better digestive function.

I recall one patient who didn't respond to any changes in diet or supplements over several consultations. We had established a good rapport, and I had a hunch and asked her, 'What's eating you up?' There was an awkward silence, then she burst into tears as she confessed an act of infidelity several years previously in her otherwise good marriage. After that, her IBS cleared up.

With so many possible triggers of IBS, care needs to be taken in formulating a treatment programme on the understanding that no two people are the same. It's important to investigate the underlying factors for each individual and deal with these, rather than simply treating the symptoms.

A majority of IBS sufferers find that increasing soluble fibre helps enormously, especially for those with constipation. Fibre not only helps make bowel movements more regular in the short term, but also tones the intestinal muscles, keeps the gut lining cleaner, and helps to balance the gut flora, but the type of fibre used is important. Wheat bran, a popular choice, can sometimes do more harm than good, not just because wheat itself is a common allergen but also because the bran actually irritates the intestinal lining. Fruit and vegetable fibre, on the other hand, as well as other grains (such as brown rice, rye and quinoa) can benefit many people with IBS. People with diarrhoea must be careful, as some fibre might aggravate them – pectin (apples, bananas) and algin (seaweeds) may be helpful. If you increase the fibre in your diet, it is important also to drink more water.

Some people, however, are extremely sensitive to any fibre-rich foods and do better on a FODMAP diet.

Alongside a wholefood diet free from refined foods, there are several supplements – vitamins, minerals, essential fats, amino acids, herbs and other botanical preparations – that can help immensely. Supporting the liver with these is also an important part of the cleansing and healing process (see Chapter 25). Vitamin B complex, for example, is needed for proper muscle tone, for the absorption of foods, for repair, for metabolising foods and generally in our response to stress. Magnesium can help reduce muscle spasms, as can peppermint oil, as mentioned earlier.

A clinical nutritionist can help you identify which

supplements will best suit your individual needs and can advise you on lifestyle practices that can help to alleviate IBS. The symptoms of IBS can be overcome by diet, supplements, exercise and relaxation, and although the underlying causes and correct treatment might take a while to unravel, it can ultimately allow most people who have IBS to lead fulfilling, active lives.

Summary – Chapter 23

To identify and treat the underlying causes of IBS, as well as experience relief from associated symptoms or conditions, it is worth considering the following lifestyle and dietary factors:

- Prior to any treatment of suspected IBS, check with your practitioner regarding any other underlying conditions that could potentially be associated to your symptoms.
- It is worth confirming, via a stool analysis, if you have a bacterial imbalance.
- Follow the dietary tips and behavioural therapies provided in this chapter.
- If experiencing excessive flatulence, try the FODMAP diet for one week. Alternatively, avoid the food you react to and supplement probiotics.
- For those experiencing associated ANS reactions, consume anti-inflammatory foods or try supplementing an enteric-coated peppermint oil capsule (an anti-spasmodic, natural treatment), 3 times a day.

- Supplementing magnesium, vitamin B complex, zinc, vitamin A, essential fats and glutamine can contribute to gut healing. If supplementing prebiotics, ensure you do not have SIBO, as this can lead to microbial overgrowth.

CHAPTER 24

How to Beat Candida

One of the most common gastrointestinal infections is called candidiasis, otherwise known as yeast infection. This is an overgrowth of a common intestinal yeast, *Candida albicans*, which normally resides in the large intestine but can migrate into the small intestine and put down roots. The name *Candida albicans* means 'sweet and white', suggesting something delicate and pure, but in reality *C. albicans* is a minute microbe, a yeast, which multiplies, migrates and releases toxins. As a result, it can afflict us with countless symptoms, both physical and mental – bowel problems, allergies, hormone dysfunction, skin complaints, joint and muscle pain, thrush, infections, ear and sinus problems, emotional disorders and fatigue – many of which mimic other diseases and are frequently misdiagnosed. A common complaint from people with candidiasis is that they feel ill all over.

Many people who suffer at the hands of this microbe personify candida as an enemy with which they must engage in long and determined warfare. The only certain way to victory is to understand its tactics and take the offensive with all guns blazing. This enemy will lose no opportunity to regain lost ground, so the battle must be unrelenting until at last it is won – and even then there is the danger of a false treaty.

This distressing situation is largely human made, however: we eat an incredible amount of sugar, which nourishes our resident yeast; refined grains such as white flour and white rice quickly convert to glucose when digested, adding to the body's sugar load; antibiotics used indiscriminately reduce friendly bacteria and create more room in the intestines for yeast and other pathogenic microbes; steroid drugs and hormone treatments depress the immune system so that it cannot effectively fight back at invading pathogens; the formulae in babies' bottles ensure an early imbalance in bowel ecology; and stress – even just the daily stress of modern life – triggers the release of the body's sugar stores, providing yet another source of nourishment for yeast. Candida cannot take all the blame; we give it every encouragement. The first stage in fighting back is therefore to start taking personal responsibility for our health.

Obviously, it is important to ensure that the enemy is correctly identified. Back in 1983, Dr William Crook published a questionnaire in his book, *The Yeast Connection*, to help ascertain the presence or severity of an overgrowth of candida. If the responses to the questionnaire showed a high score, and if doctors had failed to make any other diagnosis, the questionnaire indicated that it would make sense to embark on an anti-candida campaign with the support of a clinical nutritionist. A questionnaire showing historical predisposing factors and current symptoms is probably still the most reliable tool for indicating the presence of an overgrowth of yeast. The following questions have been adapted and designed to help you discover your own potential for candidiasis, although a nutritional therapist can also test for an overgrowth of candida in the gut and the presence of anti-candida antibodies. I recommend having a test if you score positive on the basis of symptoms.

The candida questionnaire –
how do you score?

History:
Score 2 points for each 'yes' answer in this section.

1. Have you taken tetracycline or other antibiotics for one month or longer? ☐
2. Have you, at any time in your life, taken other 'broad spectrum' antibiotics for respiratory, urinary or other infections (for two months or longer, or in shorter courses four or more times in a one-year period)? ☐
3. Have you, at any time in your life, been bothered by persistent prostatitis, vaginitis or other problems affecting your reproductive organs? ☐
4. Have you taken birth-control pills for more than six months? ☐
5. Have you taken steroid medication or non-steroidal anti-inflammatory drugs for more than a month? ☐

Symptoms:
Score 2 points for each 'yes' answer in this section.

1. Does exposure to perfumes, cigarette smoke, or garden or household chemicals provoke noticeable symptoms? ☐
2. Are your symptoms worse on damp, muggy days or in mouldy places? ☐
3. Do you have athlete's foot, ringworm, 'jock itch' or other chronic fungal infections of the skin or nails? ☐
4. Do you crave sugar, bread, cheese or alcoholic beverages? ☐

Now score 1 point for each symptom in the questions that follow (for example, the first question score could be 0, 1, 2 or 3):

1. Do you often experience fatigue, lethargy or drowsiness? (The top score could be 3.) ☐
2. Do you ever have the feeling of being 'drained'? ☐
3. Do you suffer from depression or anxiety? (The top score could be 2.) ☐
4. Do you have poor memory?` ☐
5. Do you ever experience feeling 'spacey'? ☐
6. Do you suffer from an inability to concentrate or difficulty in making decisions? (The top score could be 2.) ☐
7. Do you experience numbness, burning, tingling or itching? (The top score could be 4.) ☐
8. Do you ever get headaches, migraines, sinusitis or nasal congestion? (The top score could be 4.) ☐
9. Do you suffer from muscle aches or muscle weakness? (The top score could be 2.) ☐
10. Do you have painful joints or swelling in the joints? (The top score could be 2.) ☐
11. Do you suffer from abdominal pain? ☐
12. Do you get constipation and/or diarrhoea? (The top score could be 2.) ☐
13. Do you suffer from bloating, belching, 'wind', indigestion, or heartburn? (The top score could be 5.) ☐
14. Do you have vaginal burning, itching or discharge? (The top score could be 3.) ☐
15. Do you suffer from prostatitis, impotence or infertility? (The top score could be 3.) ☐
16. Do you ever experience a loss of sexual desire? ☐

17. Do you have menstrual pain or irregularities, endometriosis or infertility? (The top score could be 4.) ☐
18. Do you get premenstrual symptoms such as headaches, irritability, depression, bloating, tiredness, tender breasts? (The top score could be 6). ☐
19. Do you ever have urinary frequency, urgency or burning? (The top score could be 3.) ☐
20. Do you suffer from cold hands or feet and/or general chilliness? (The top score could be 2.) ☐
21. Do you suffer from irritability or jitteriness? (The top score could be 2.) ☐
22. Do you have persistent acne, eczema or psoriasis? (The top score could be 3.) ☐

Add up your **total score**. ☐

Male: If you score above 45, there's a strong likelihood that you have candidiasis. If you score above 30 there's a possibility that you have a degree of candidiasis.

Female: If you score above 55, there's a strong likelihood that you have candidiasis. If you score above 35 there's a possibility that you have a degree of candidiasis.

If you score above these levels, I recommend that you see a nutritional therapist to investigate the situation and advise you appropriately.

The anti-candida four-point plan

The four-point plan for beating candida is based on a diet that first starves the organism; you then supplement natural anti-candida agents, boost your immune system and restore healthy gut bacteria.

1 Diet

The aim of the diet is to starve candida to death. As sugar encourages yeast to overgrow and become an invading fungus, all forms of it must be strictly avoided. The most obvious form of sugar is sucrose, which means avoiding all sweetened cakes, biscuits and confectionery (including chocolate). Lactose (milk sugar) is also effective at encouraging candida, which means that cow's milk and cheese must be avoided. (For some people, it is possible to have natural yoghurt, cottage cheese and butter; this depends on various factors, including the possibility of dairy intolerance.) Fructose (fruit sugar) provides another form of nourishment for candida, which means that all fruit has to be avoided. Refined carbohydrates add to the glucose load, so it is essential to use only wholegrain flour, rice, etc. Other substances to be avoided are yeast (bread, gravy mixes, spreads), fermented products (alcohol, vinegar), mould (cheese, mushrooms), and stimulants (tea, coffee). Various additives also need to be avoided, in particular monosodium glutamate (produced by fermentation) and citric acid (produced by adding sugar to mould). At first glance, it might seem that there is nothing left to eat. In fact, there is a very great deal which can still be enjoyed, and a positive approach to the diet is essential. I recommend that you read *The Beat Candida Cookbook* by Erica White, which demonstrates that mealtimes can still be an enjoyable experience.

There is some debate regarding xylitol, a sugar alcohol that stops bacteria sticking to things. Apart from being extremely low GL, the *Candida albicans* organism cannot live off it in the same ways it does off sugar.

Case Study: Charles

Charles, who had suffered from chronic candidiasis for over 10 years, shared this:

'Being a fruit lover who used to eat lots of fruit on a daily basis, I started looking for a safe way to have sweet stuff without feeding the microorganisms that have been for so long attacking my system. After lengthy research taking more than a year, I found out that although most sweeteners feed bacteria and *Candida albicans*, xylitol does not. I started using xylitol regularly and found out, to my surprise, that my worst candida symptoms were gone. The symptoms would recur every time I had fruits (darn!) or something made with refined sugar or other sweeteners like Splenda or stevia, or even the aspartame that is used in diet drinks. Whether I liked it or not, it became clear to me that I could not eat or drink anything sweet, that I could neither have any fruits nor drink any diet sodas. I have intensely and extensively 'tested' xylitol for over a year and I can affirm without a doubt that it is the only sweetener I can use without getting my symptoms back.'

Even so, I would use xylitol in small quantities and with caution. This is uncharted territory.

Candida often triggers cravings for its favourite foods, so at these times steely determination is needed to keep to the anti-candida diet. Temporary help might be obtained from an amino acid supplement, L-glutamine, which can help to block the cravings and make it easier to get established on the diet. Your motivation will be encouraged if you have a clear understanding of what is happening, and before long a 'sweet tooth' will disappear, making it easier to stay on a sugar-free diet. Even when candida-related symptoms have completely disappeared, the diet should be maintained for a further year in order to consolidate the newly corrected balance of gut flora. Most people are more than happy to do this because they so much appreciate their restored health.

2 Your personal supplement programme

A supplement programme must be devised to help strengthen immunity, to correct imbalances in glucose tolerance, hormonal status and histamine levels, and to detoxify the body of pollutants. It is important to support the immune system in as many ways as possible in order to fight back against candida. An appropriate supplement programme can be formulated through an analysis of your symptoms, which will give strong pointers to your nutritional deficiencies and imbalances. Ideally, your nutritional status should be monitored and the supplement programme reassessed at three-monthly intervals. My 100% Health Check can work this out for you (see Resources).

In an otherwise carefully calculated programme of nutrients, vitamin C can be taken to bowel tolerance levels (the amount just below that which causes loose bowels) to help rid the body of toxins.

3 Anti-fungal supplements

One of the most useful anti-fungal agents is **caprylic acid**, a fatty acid that occurs naturally in coconuts. Its great advantages are that it does not adversely affect beneficial organisms and it is fat-soluble so it is able to penetrate cell membranes. Taken as calcium/magnesium caprylate, it survives the digestive processes and is able to reach the colon. For reasons yet to be discussed, it is essential to start with a low level and build up slowly, a process facilitated by capsules of different strengths.

Grapefruit seed extract has powerful properties that are antibiotic, anti-fungal and anti-viral. Like caprylic acid, one of its great advantages is that it has little adverse effect on the beneficial gut bacteria. It can be taken in capsules or as drops, again starting at a low level and increasing very gradually. It is thought to be more gentle on the intestinal lining than caprylic acid, so should be considered when there is a history of gastrointestinal inflammation such as ulceration, gastritis or colitis. (However, no type of anti-fungal should be taken while any of these conditions still persist, and neither should they be taken during pregnancy.)

Oregano oil Caprylic acid and grapefruit seed extract are frequently followed by oregano oil. Its structure makes it better able to penetrate the gut wall, so it can be useful for symptoms in parts of the body away from the gastrointestinal tract, for example the joints, skin and sinuses. Capsules should be started at 1 daily and increased (as symptoms allow) to 2 daily. Oregano oil should not be taken with certain health conditions, so you should consult a nutritional therapist.

Olive leaf extract is potent and therefore likely to give rise to a strong die-off reaction (see page 263). For this reason, it is frequently introduced as the final anti-fungal approach when gut ecology has almost reached its equilibrium. As usual, the capsules should be started at 1 daily and increased only gradually.

Propolis is another natural substance which, according to research at the University of Bratislava, is remarkably effective for all fungal infections of the skin and body. It can be taken as drops and built up gradually. Its anaesthetic effect is soothing for oral thrush, and as cream, for painful muscles and fungal nails.

Aloe vera is gently anti-fungal and is a refreshing mouthwash or gargle as well as an aid to digestion. It can be used as an overnight denture soak, preferable to products that are not specifically anti-fungal. Dentures can be an ongoing source of candida re-infection; however, it is very important to find a product that does not contain citric acid.

Tea tree oil is an anti-fungal agent and, as a cream, can be used for fungal skin conditions. Candida is frequently associated with eczema, psoriasis and acne as well as athlete's foot and other fungal skin or nail infections. **Herbal chickweed** ointment can be helpful for reducing irritation.

Sometimes, in addition to a range of candida-related symptoms, persistent low body weight and diarrhoea might suggest a gut parasite infection, in which case it can be helpful to have a parasitology laboratory test. A nutritional therapist can then decide on an appropriate anti-fungal, anti-parasitic supplement. It is still necessary to monitor intake of anti-candida agents so that die-off reaction of the candida is kept to a minimum. (Die-off occurs as toxins are released from the dead candida. With this release there is a general feeling of unwellness and what might appear as a flare-up of old symptoms. I explain the die-off reaction in detail on page 263.)

As surprising as it might sound, one of the best supplements to tackle candida is itself a yeast, called *Saccharomyces boulardii*.[88] It's a non-colonising yeast, which means that it will never take up residence in your gut. As it passes through, it stimulates your gut's production of the immune component secretory immunoglobulin A (SIgA). Greater amounts of this immunoglobulin make it increasingly difficult for the candida to stick to your gut wall. Some people with candida might be hypersensitive to all yeast including *S. boulardii*, so taking it could make you feel worse. In which case, you should wait until you've cut all yeast out of your diet for about four weeks to reduce your hypersensitivity and then introduce the *S. boulardii* at very low doses and increase it very gradually. This might mean starting with as little as 1 billion organisms (½ capsule) once daily before building up to the full dose of about 10 billion organisms a day. *S. boulardii* also helps to make the environment of your gut more hospitable to friendly bacteria, thereby enhancing their chances of taking up residence.

You can take the other anti-candida agents – caprylic acid, oregano oil and olive leaf extract – while you are taking *S. boulardii*, but they should be taken several hours apart so as not to kill off the *S. boulardii* as well. It's generally best not to start any of these additional supplements until you've been on the anti-candida diet and have been taking the *S. boulardii* for about a month in order to minimise the die-off reaction.

4 Probiotics

Supplements are needed to carry beneficial bacteria into the intestines to re-establish a healthy colony. The Americans call it 're-florestation'! The role of these bifidobacteria is to increase acidity by producing lactic acid and acetic acid, and to inhibit undesirable microorganisms that would compete against them for attachment sites. Tissues densely covered with beneficial organisms provide an effective blocking mechanism against invading pathogens (rather like a flower-bed packed with plants allows little room for weeds to grow).

Lactobacillus acidophilus is the major coloniser of the small intestine and *Bifidobacterium bifidum* inhabits the large intestine (where it produces B vitamins) and the vagina. Other helpful bacteria are the transient *Lactobacillus bulgaricus* and *Streptococcus thermophilus*, which produce lactic acid as they pass through the bowel. These friendly bacteria are contained in live natural yoghurt, which is therefore a helpful food provided you have no intolerance to dairy products. In live yoghurt, the lactose (milk sugar) content has largely been converted into lactic acid by enzyme-producing bifidobacteria, which accounts for the sharpness of its taste. To understand more about these bacteria read Chapter 7.

To ensure safe passage of these bacteria through the gastric juices, it is necessary to take them in a capsule supplying large numbers of viable organisms in freeze-dried form. Two capsules should be taken daily with food but away from anti-fungals. This level needs to be increased only in cases of diarrhoea or following antibiotics, which further deplete the bifidobacteria. An *acidophilus* cream is a beneficial aid for a vaginal fungal infection.

That is the anti-candida four-point plan, which has been effective for countless people. Each of the four points is essential in the fight against candida. Non-compliance with any one of them will almost certainly lead to failure. There is also a fifth vital aspect: support. Anyone entering this war zone will almost certainly find themselves in a minefield of problems. Confusion and depression are common, and someone is needed who can look at the situation objectively, discern what is happening and point the way forward. This is part of the role of a supportive nutritional therapist.

How to deal with die-off

Thriving candida is known to release a minimum of 79 toxins. Dead candida is known to release even more. A general feeling of toxicity includes aching muscles, fuzzy head, depression, anxiety, itching, nausea and diarrhoea. In addition, in specific areas where candida has colonised, there is likely to be an apparent flare-up of old symptoms, such as sore throat, thrush, painful joints, eczema, and so on. This unpleasant situation is known as 'die-off' or more formally as 'Herxheimer reaction'. It needs to be recognised as a last-ditch deception by the enemy, because the very presence of die-off symptoms means that candida is being wiped out and that victory is imminent. Unfortunately, many people have not been forewarned of this, and in consequence they misinterpret the situation by deciding that the anti-candida diet or the supplements are making them even more ill so, not surprisingly, they give up the programme – which sadly means that they have taken a big step backwards. Forewarned is very definitely forearmed!

The art of destroying candida is to do so slowly but surely so that it is not killed off faster than the body can eliminate the extra toxins. Initial die-off is usually triggered by the diet as candida is starved to death and also by vitamins and minerals as they boost the immune system to fight more strongly. These first two points of the four-point plan usually cause more than enough die-off for most people to cope with, and anti-fungal agents should not be added to the regime until this phase is over. By the end of a month the majority of people claim that they feel better than they have for years and are ready to start anti-fungal and probiotic supplements – although die-off is still likely to occur as anti-fungals are first introduced and then increased, which explains why it is important to increase them slowly and gradually.

Taking ground slowly is the surest method of attack. Most people starting on caprylic acid can tolerate one medium-strength capsule (400mg) daily, without too much difficulty. If, after a week, they are not battling with die-off symptoms, the dose can be increased to 2 × 400mg, and so on, up to six capsules daily, but increasing only as die-off symptoms allow – which might sometimes mean staying at a certain level for two weeks or even longer. After this, they can grad-uate to 3 × 680mg capsules and increase again, taking it as slowly as necessary. The climb up is seldom straightforward, and at some stage there might come a surge of die-off reaction necessitating a drop to a lower level, or even a complete break from anti-fungals, while the body eliminates the toxins. This should not be regarded as a setback, but simply as a necessary part of the process. Drinking plenty of fluid and taking good levels of vitamin C will speed up the body's detoxification, but at the same time it is wise to support the liver while it undertakes this additional work. Taking herbal supplements of milk thistle (silymarin) can be beneficial, and drinking several cups daily of dandelion root 'coffee' increases the pro-duction of bile, which carries toxins out of the liver.

Sometimes, the worst die-off related symptom to bear is an increase in anxiety or depression. This is thought to be caused by an immune reaction to die-off toxins, in other words an allergic reaction to the toxins, making die-off twice as bad as it would otherwise be. In this situation, a nutritional therapist can assess the situation and suggest supplements to help moderate the symptoms.

Eventually, the anti-fungal supplements accomplish their work, indicated by a sense of well-being that is confirmed by a drop in the candida score to its lowest possible level (allowing for 'history' factors, which obviously do not change).

When progress appears to be slow, this might be due to environmental factors (such as inhaling domestic gas or even mould from house-plant soil), or to unsuspected food sensitivities that are overloading the immune system. Avoidance of culprit foods, best tested with an IgG food intolerance test (see Resources) enables the immune system to strengthen its fight against candida. Discovering environmental culprits involves detection and possibly expense if, for example, the heating system needs to be changed from gas to electricity! Much more often, though, it's just a case of finding temporary foster homes for beloved house plants. It really does make a tremendous difference to get air-borne mould spores from damp soil out of your home.

Having said this, it's an unfortunate fact that, when allergens such as mould are removed, there is likely to be a surge of die-off symptoms. This is because a load has been removed from the immune system, enabling it to destroy candida more efficiently. During this phase it is best to have a break from anti-fungal supplements because enough is happening – and it's essential to remember that die-off is a 'good thing', because it shows that more of the candida is being destroyed.

Another block to progress can be stress, since it triggers the release of the body's sugar stores, providing nourishment for resident candida. A test for adrenal stress hormones can point to appropriate supplemental support to be introduced, thereby allowing the four-point plan to have greater success in bringing candida under control.

Read Chapter 11, and my book *The Stress Cure*, to build up your stress resilience.

Candidiasis is frequently not acknowledged or suspected by medical practitioners, and it is often misunderstood by family and friends. Consequent loneliness and despair add to the physical and mental suffering caused by candida itself. There is no easy way to win the candida war. It takes courage, determination and perseverance, but it can most certainly be done!

Summary – Chapter 24

If you do have candidiasis – which needs to be properly diagnosed based on symptoms and tests – there's a four-point plan to follow to beat candida:

- Follow a strict anti-candida diet such as that in Erica White's *Beat Candida Cookbook*. This is entirely sugar-free, including fruits.
- Build up your immunity with a personalised supplement programme (complete the 100% Health Check – see Resources).
- Take anti-fungal supplements, primarily caprylic acid in increasing doses, as well as *Saccharomyces boulardii*.
- Take probiotics, a combination of *Lactobacillus* and bifidobacteria, always away from anti-fungals.

CHAPTER 25

Liver Detoxification Problems – the Cause of Chronic Fatigue?

I f you have increased intestinal permeability, your liver will be working overtime to deal with the extra toxins, improperly digested foods and potential allergens that can get through your digestive tract into your blood. A good 80 per cent of the chemical processes that go on in the body involve detoxifying thousands of potentially harmful substances. Much of this is done by the liver, which represents a clearing house, able to recognise millions of potentially harmful chemicals and transform them into something harmless or prepare them for elimination. It assembles amino acids, stores vitamins and minerals, makes cholesterol and bile, controls glucose and fat supplies, balances hormones and plays a key role in immunity. It is the chemical brain of the body – recycling, regenerating and detoxifying in order to maintain your health.

Most of us tend to assume that food is always good for us. Of course it is, but the truth is that almost all food contains toxins as well as nutrients. So too do air and water. These external toxins, or exotoxins, are just a small part of what the liver has to deal with; many toxins are made by the body from otherwise harmless molecules. Every thought, every breath and every action generate toxins. These internally created toxins, or endotoxins, have to be disarmed in just the same way as exotoxins. Whether a substance is bad for you or not depends as much on your ability to detoxify it as on its inherent toxic properties. People with multiple food sensitivities are eating the same food as healthy people – they have just lost their ability to detoxify it.

Instead of thinking of certain substances as 'bad' for you, or provoking allergies, think of them as exceeding your adaptive capacity. It's as if the body's metabolism represents a fire. The fire generates smoke that needs to be got rid of. Our metabolic fire (the consequence of releasing the energy from the sun stored in plants that we eat and 'combust') generates plenty of 'smoke', or oxidants. That's what the liver has to deal with. It's the 'smoke', not the substances themselves, that often causes problems.

Detoxification – a two-step process

The way the liver detoxifies this smoke can be split into two stages.

Phase 1 is akin to getting your rubbish ready for collection. It doesn't actually eliminate anything, it just prepares it for elimination, making it easier to pick up. Fat-soluble toxins, for example, become more soluble.

Phase 1 is carried out by a series of enzymes called P-450 enzymes. The more toxins you're exposed to, the faster these enzymes must work to pile up the rubbish ready for collection. Often, the substances created by the P-450 enzyme reactions are more toxic than before; for example, many are oxidised, generating harmful free radicals. The function of P-450 enzymes depends on a long list of nutrients, including vitamins B_2, B_3, B_6, B_{12}, folic acid, glutathione, amino acids (leucine, isoleucine, valine), flavonoids and phospholipids, plus a generous supply of antioxidant nutrients to deal with the oxidants. A person who has a high exposure to toxins (due to diet and lifestyle factors or digestive problems) may have a revved up Phase 1, used to working hard and fast to get these toxins ready for collection. Substances that get Phase 1 going include caffeine, alcohol, dioxins, cigarette smoke, exhaust fumes, high-protein diets, organophosphate fertilisers, paint fumes, saturated fat, steroid hormones and charcoal-barbecued meat.

Phase 2 This next stage is more about building up than breaking down. The end-products of Phase 1 are transformed by 'sticking' things on to them in a process called 'conjugation' in order to make them easier to dispose of. Some toxins have glutathione stuck to them (this is 'glutathione conjugation'). This is how we detoxify paracetamol (acetaminophen), for example. In cases of overdose, a person is given glutathione to mop up the highly destructive toxins generated by Phase 1 detoxification of this drug.

Other toxins have sulphur stuck to them in a process called 'sulphation'. This is the fate of many steroid hormones, neurotransmitters and, once again, paracetamol. The sulphur comes directly from food. Garlic, onions and eggs are good sources of sulphur-containing amino acids, such as methionine and cysteine, so if you lack these in

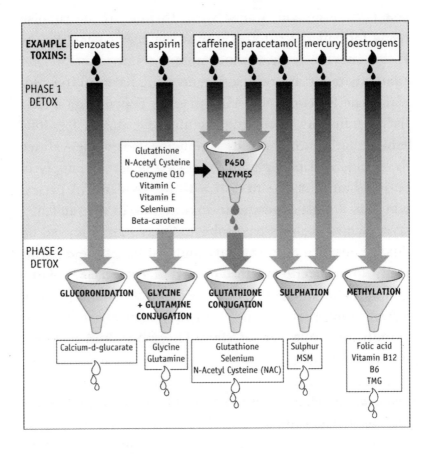

The key detox nutrients your liver needs

your diet, you've got a problem with sulphation. Other toxins have carbon compounds, called methyl groups, stuck to them (this is called 'methylation'). Lead and arsenic are detoxified in this way. Aspirin has the amino acid glycine stuck to it (this is called 'glycine conjugation'). When these pathways are overloaded, the body can use another, known as glucuronidation, which is the primary route for breaking down many tranquillisers.

Too many toxins – or not enough nutrients?

When these biochemical pathways don't work properly, due to an overload or a lack of nutrients, the body generates harmful toxins. An example is homocysteine, a toxic by-product of breaking down the amino acid methionine. This can be a result of problems with sulphation (usually due to a lack of vitamin B_6) or methylation (which involves folic acid and B_{12}). Sulphur dioxide, a component of exhaust fumes, is detoxified via the sulphation pathway, whose enzymes depend on the mineral molybdenum, which is found in particularly high amounts in beans. Overexposure, coupled with a molybdenum-deficient diet, can lead to an intolerance of exhaust fumes.

Both phases of detoxifying pathways work together. If one is overloaded, a toxin might be processed by another. Homocysteine can, as a back-up, be mopped up by glycine conjugation, which is why taking in more of the amino acid glycine often has the effect of lowering an elevated homocysteine level.

Liver problems or health problems?

Taking a liver's view of disease processes often sheds new light on some common health problems of the twenty-first century; for example, just about any allergic, inflammatory or metabolic disorder, including eczema, asthma, chronic fatigue, chronic infections, inflammatory bowel disorders, multiple sclerosis, rheumatoid arthritis, and even schizophrenia and hormone imbalances, may involve or create sub-optimum liver function.

Many hormone-related problems in women are currently blamed on 'oestrogen dominance'. The body makes oestrogen and maintains the right balance by a series of processes in the liver. The balance of oestrone, oestradiol and oestriol (the three oestrogenic hormones) is critical to health. The transformation of one into another and their degradation are controlled by the liver.

Poor liver function, then, can lead to an imbalance and accumulation of oestrogenic hormones.

The liver is also the buffer for too much glucose in the blood, converting it into fat. But it has a limit and the excess fat spills over into the liver, creating fatty liver disease.

The brain is not able to disarm a wide range of toxins – it depends on the liver to do a chemical clean-up of the blood before it gets there. An example is alcohol. Once you start to get drunk you've exceeded the liver's capacity to detoxify alcohol.

Toxic overload of the liver has dire consequences for brain and nervous-system function. Autism, schizophrenia and memory loss are all associated with poor liver function. A classic example is alcoholism. When the liver can't deal with the quantity of alcohol consumed, the brain is left unprotected. This is why brain damage, dementia and mental illness are some particularly unpleasant consequences of chronic alcohol abuse.

If you drink too much alcohol, the liver generates increased levels of acetaldehyde, which is what causes a hangover. Curcumin, the active ingredient in turmeric, supplemented in sufficient quantities or in a highly absorbable form called theracurmin, has been shown to dramatically reduce levels of acetaldehyde.[89]

Cholesterol and blood sugar control

Cholesterol is a major building block for hormones. Your body can use it to make the sex hormones testosterone, oestrogen and progesterone as well as adrenal hormones. Cholesterol is both made and detoxified by the liver. If you need more, it will make it. If you need less, it will break it down – if it can.

From cholesterol, the liver can make bile to digest fat. The body makes no less than 1 litre of bile each day. Although most is reabsorbed from the digestive tract into the blood, the small amount that leaves the body takes with it toxins excreted by the liver. Liver problems usually lead to an accumulation of fat in the liver which can be responsible for 'fatty liver' or 'sluggish liver', associated with excess alcohol and sugar consumption, since the liver has to convert excess into fat for storage.

The liver can also turn sugar into glycogen and fat. When your blood sugar level is low, it turns glycogen back into glucose. By ensuring optimal liver function, you improve your body's ability to maintain the correct balance of cholesterol, triglycerides (blood fats) and glucose, which are vital to maintaining good health.

Gall bladder problems and gall stones

If your liver isn't working properly, you can form gallstones in the gall bladder, which can measure up to 5cm across. If a stone becomes lodged in the bile duct – the tube from the gall bladder to the duodenum – you will experience excruciating pain. There are two main types of gallstones, although you can have a combination of both. The more common type is primarily composed of cholesterol and is yellow/green in colour. Other stones are brown in colour, composed mainly of bilirubin, calcium and salts. These types can be ultrasonically broken up. However, the most usual treatment is removal of the gall bladder.

If you've had your gall bladder removed, the liver still produces bile, but it's not nearly as concentrated and isn't automatically released when you eat fat. This means that you can still digest some fat but not so much, so it is important to eat a consistently low-fat diet. One way to improve matters is to supplement lecithin with any meal containing fat, as lecithin is the main emulsifying agent that prepares fat for digestion. Lecithin is available either as granules (in which case you simply add a dessertspoonful to each meal) or as capsules (in which case you take 1,200mg with each meal). You can also assist fat digestion by taking a digestive enzyme containing lipase.

Testing for liver function

Standard tests for liver function involve measuring levels of the key enzymes GPT (glutamate-pyruvate transaminase) and GOT (glutamate-oxaloacetate transaminase). If they are raised, it means your liver is struggling. This is an indication of a chronic problem and, although it is useful in pinpointing that a problem exists, it doesn't really identify the best way to help recovery.

A more advanced and detailed indication of liver function, capable of picking up imbalances before they develop into chronic health problems, is a comprehensive detoxification profile. This is a non-invasive test that involves ingesting a measured amount of caffeine, aspirin and paracetamol and then analysing certain chemicals that appear in the urine. How these substances are dealt with and what they turn into helps determine which pathways are working and which ones aren't. If one pathway is underfunctioning, another might be overfunctioning to help cope with the load.

Some people with toxic overload – perhaps from over-exposure to exotoxins, or a gut infection in which the disease-causing organism generates toxins, or a leaky gut in which toxic substances are more easily able to enter the body – become 'pathological detoxifiers'. This means their Phase 1 system is hyperactive, trying to get the endless rubbish ready for collection. Phase 2 processes, meanwhile, are overloaded and simply can't deal with all the toxins being generated. In these cases, just giving a person a lot of B vitamins could make them worse, not better, because these nutrients further speed up Phase 1, thus increasing the overload on the Phase 2 processes.

Chronic fatigue solutions

One of the consequences of poor liver function is chronic fatigue. By now it will be no surprise to find that poor nutrition, poor digestion, dysbiosis, gut inflammation and a leaky gut can all contribute to chronic fatigue. These factors are very rarely checked and corrected in orthodox medical treatment of chronic fatigue syndrome (CFS) which has only recently been accepted as a true disease state.

Research by Dr Jeffrey Bland and colleagues at the US Institute of Functional Medicine tested 30 CFS patients for liver detoxification abnormalities and then devised a nutritional strategy designed to correct these. Using their

Metabolic Screening Questionnaire the initial symptom score over the 21 days of the study dropped by more than half; this was consistent with improvements shown by further liver-function tests.[90]

In later research, they identified that a significant proportion of CFS patients show a particular type of imbalance in liver detoxification in which the first phase is very speedy, generating toxins, while the second phase is sluggish, resulting in an inability to clear those toxins.[91] With this in mind, it's a good idea for people with CFS to have their liver function assessed and treated using specifically designed nutritional support.

Other factors that might be involved are food allergies and intolerances (often the consequence of leaky gut syndrome), adrenal exhaustion, thyroid problems and blood sugar imbalances.

A key focus for new research has been looking at how the body's mitochondria – the tiny engines within each of our cells that make energy – can become deficient. These microscopic powerhouses are necessary for every bodily function, and if they malfunction, the result is extreme fatigue.

Dr Sarah Myhill, a GP who specialises in treating CFS, has pioneered research in this area and has treated hundreds of sufferers successfully. Her approach addresses many of the areas outlined earlier; but, crucially, she also assesses for mitochondrial dysfunction, which appears to be a common feature in all CFS sufferers, no matter what other underlying causes exist.

In the past few years, a new test has been developed which makes it possible to measure mitochondrial dysfunction, and also to assess which of the many nutrients necessary for energy production in the mitochondria are in short supply. Interestingly, magnesium is one such key nutrient, which might explain why earlier research often found CFS sufferers to be deficient in magnesium. But co-enzyme Q_{10}, B_3 (niacin) and acetyl L-carnitine are also important.

In a study of 138 patients with CFS conducted by Dr Myhill and Professor Norman Booth of Oxford University, mitochondrial dysfunction was indeed identified in every single case.[92] They also found that the level of dysfunction correlated to the degree of fatigue experienced. As Dr Myhill observed, 'These patients do not suffer from hypochondria – the problem is mitochondria,' which must have been a great relief to sufferers who are likely to have been dismissed by others in the medical profession.

Restoring optimal liver function

The good news is that, with a good diet, lifestyle and the right supplements, you can restore your health, improve your digestion, get your mitochondria working properly and maintain optimal liver function. For people with long-term health problems, especially those involving chronic fatigue, allergies, chemical sensitivities or digestive disorders, it is well worth seeing a clinical nutritionist and having the necessary tests. He or she can help to identify the sources of toxic overload and recommend how to eliminate them. They can also recommend the correct balance of nutrients to get the liver's log-jam moving again, if that is your problem. For personal guidance and referral for a Comprehensive Detoxification Profile, you should consult a clinical nutritional therapist (see Resources).

Prevention, however, is better than cure, so if you are basically healthy and want to promote and maintain optimal liver function, the best advice is to cut down on your intake of toxic substances, eat an optimal diet and follow a balanced nutrition supplement programme. In practice, this means you should:

- Minimise your intake of alcohol, caffeine, cigarettes, sugar, fried foods, saturated fat, pesticides, exhaust fumes and medications.
- Eat a low-GL diet – high blood sugar is a major cause of liver stress.
- Increase your intake of all fruits and vegetables, especially those rich in antioxidants (carrots, tomatoes, green peppers, watercress, and so on), anthocyanidins (berries, beetroot, grapes), and glucosinolates (cabbage, broccoli, Brussels sprouts, kale). Eat carnivorous fish, high in omega-3, in place of meat, and cold-pressed seeds and seed oils instead of butter; and drink plenty of purified water. Artichokes and turmeric also aid liver function.
- Supplement a high-strength multivitamin–mineral, additional antioxidant nutrients and at least 2,000mg of vitamin C per day. Some supplement companies also produce specific nutrient combinations designed to support liver function. Nutrients that can specifically help the liver are choline, methionine, liver extract and the herbs turmeric (contains curcumin), milk thistle (contains silymarin) and dandelion root.

To give your liver a complete tune up, see my book *9-Day Liver Detox Diet*, and also take the recommended supplements.

Summary – Chapter 25

To improve your liver's detoxification potential and maintain optimal digestion and liver function I would recommend:

- If you are suffering from allergic, inflammatory, hormonal and metabolic disorders, consult your health practitioner to test your liver enzymes as this will give you an insight into how well your liver is functioning.
- If your gall bladder has been removed, support your bile production by adhering to a low-fat diet, and/or supplementing a spoonful of lecithin granules per meal or 1,200mg if in the form of capsules per meal. Alternatively, supplement the digestive enzyme lipase.
- Suspected mitochondrial dysfunction linked to liver function and CFS may be corrected by supplementing a formula containing magnesium, co-enzyme Q_{10}, B_3 (niacin) and acetyl L-carnitine.
- Avoid supplementing with B vitamins if your liver is overexposed to exotoxins and is unable to detoxify them.
- Consider the recommendations on exotoxin exposure, dietary and supplement factors provided in this chapter.

CHAPTER 26

Solve Constipation, Diverticulitis and Haemorrhoids

T he single most common digestive complaint of all is constipation. It affects one in six people[93] and can be a source of considerable discomfort. To put this in context, in the US there are about 10 million visits to doctors every year for constipation-related concerns. Of these, about a quarter include other symptoms of IBS. Many of these people will receive medication of one sort or another.[94]

Constipation

Despite the high numbers given above, many more people are actually constipated without even knowing it. Ideally, you should defecate at least once a day, if not two or even three times a day, without effort or straining. In the 100% Health Survey of over 55,000 people, 83 per cent did not defecate every day. That means that more than eight in ten people had some degree of constipation. Heavy, sinking stools means your faecal matter is packed hard together, which is what the Latin verb *constipare* means. As a consequence, this puts a strain on the muscles of the colon, which can lead to colitis and diverticulitis, and a strain on the rectum, potentially causing haemorrhoids. You might also be more prone to blockages in the appendix, leading to appendicitis. Constipation also slows down the time food spends in the digestive tract, which allows more opportunity for putrefaction and exposure to toxic material. This is a major contributor to colorectal cancer and it is therefore no surprise to find that there is an association between constipation and increased risk of colorectal cancer.[95]

Constipation has many causes, the most common of which is hard faecal matter. If you eat enough soluble fibre (see Chapter 6) and have healthy bacteria, the excretion of which makes up a large part of stools, your stools should be loosely formed, perhaps breaking up on flushing, and should also float.

Supplementing bifidobacteria has been shown to relieve constipation.[96] Probiotic-friendly drinks, such as kefir, which you can make at home (see page 387), also helps to keep you regular.

Natural foods stay soft in the digestive tract because they contain fibres that absorb water and expand. Fruits and vegetables naturally contain a lot of water in themselves. Provided they are prepared properly, whole grains, such as oats and rice, absorb water and provide watery bulk for the digestive tract. Given that we are literally 65 per cent water, it makes sense to eat foods with a high water content. Meats, cheese, eggs, refined grains and wheat (because of its gluten content) can all be constipating. Although it should not be necessary to add fibre to a good diet, oat fibre has particular benefits. This is naturally present in oats, which are best soaked and eaten cold. Some foods and nutrients exert a mild laxative effect, such as flax seeds (which need to be ground and sprinkled on food) and chia seeds (which don't need to be ground), prunes and also vitamin C (in doses of several grams).

Not drinking sufficient water is a major cause of constipation. We need at least 1 litre, and ideally 2 litres of water a day for optimal digestive health, and this alone often relieves constipation. A colleague of mine, put in charge of a hospital, instigated a simple practice – putting a jug of water and a glass next to every hospitalised patient. As a result, there was a massive decrease in their drugs bill, the saving coming from laxatives!

With the right high-fibre diet and enough water, a person should experience the need to defecate two or three times a day, after meals. Many people suppress or ignore the natural need to go to the toilet, which, in itself, generates constipation. So, if you have the slightest urge to defecate after a meal, go for it.

Disturbances in the normal peristaltic muscle action of the bowel can also lead to constipation and a suppression of this natural reflex. This is discussed in the next chapter.

Natural laxatives

Most laxatives, even natural laxatives containing the herbs senna or cascara, are gastrointestinal irritants and, although they work, they don't really solve the underlying issue. They might be useful as an emergency measure, but it is not a good idea to be taking such remedies on a continual basis. Some remedies aimed at promoting regularity are concentrated fibre preparations containing things like bran, ispaghula, methylcellulose or sterculia. It is very important to drink plenty of water if you are taking such fibre supplements; however, as you start to change towards a high-fibre diet, they should not be necessary. My favourite super-soluble fibre in this respect is glucomannan (explained on page 52).

Alternatively, fructo-oligosaccharides (FOS), provided as a powder, work in a more beneficial way than conventional laxatives, which can make it harder to re-establish proper peristaltic muscle action. FOS are a type of complex carbohydrate that helps keep moisture in the gut and also stimulates the production of healthy bacteria. The same is true for inulin, from chicory root fibre. This keeps faecal matter softer and easier to pass along. Although results are not quite so rapid, this is a highly preferable way of reducing constipation.

Diverticulitis and colitis

Colitis means the large intestine is inflamed. Diverticulitis is a condition of the small and large intestine, in which pockets in the intestinal wall, called diverticula, become distended and are then more likely to get infected and inflamed. The condition, probably the result of not enough fibre and having poor supporting musculature, is rarely seen in primitive cultures. A more serious form of colitis, ulcerative colitis, is thought to be an autoimmune condition (see Chapter 19 for more details about this); however, it is quite likely that one leads to the other.

Increase gentle fibres and ease digestion

Both colitis and ulcerative colitis often result from eating low-fibre foods and foods that irritate the gut. These include alcohol, wheat and coffee. Fibre absorbs water, making the faecal matter less hard, more bulky and easier to pass through the body. Best in this respect are soluble fibres, which are found in very high amounts in oats, but also in flax seeds. Small seeds can get stuck in the extended diverticula, so any seeds eaten should be ground and soaked. Making porridge with ground seeds is a good way to increase its soluble fibres. Vegetable fibres are also important to include in one's diet, either steaming the vegetables or making soup. Stay away from wheat bran, however.

One of the most absorbent fibres is glucomannan fibre, from the konjac plant. Fibre powders based on glucomannan (see Resources), when taken with a large glass of water, or stirred into water to start the absorption process, can help restore normal gut peristalsis, the muscular action that passes faecal matter along.

There are a number of reasons, and foods, that can trigger bloating, which creates pressure in the inflamed colon. This can happen due to an unidentified food allergy or intolerance (see Chapter 10) or due to a lack of particular digestive enzymes; for example, the enzyme glucoamylase helps to digest carbohydrates in vegetables whereas alpha-galactosidase helps to digest carbohydrates in beans and lentils. It is very helpful to supplement a digestive enzyme formula which contains these, especially if certain foods trigger bloating or discomfort. Digestive enzymes should be taken at the start of a meal.

Re-inoculate the gut with beneficial bacteria

As we have seen throughout the book, the health of the digestive tract is dependent on having a healthy colony of beneficial bacteria. The two main families of essential bacteria are *Lactobacillus acidophilus* and bifidobacteria. It is worth supplementing these for a month to establish a healthy colony, then a good diet will 'feed' the bacteria so that there is no need to continue supplementation ad infinitum. Supplements of bifidobacteria have been shown to relieve constipation (see above). Some yoghurts use these essential strains of bacteria, but most don't. Be wary of yoghurt as a source of bacteria if you suspect you might be dairy intolerant.

Some digestive-enzyme supplements also contain beneficial bacteria as well as glutamine, an essential amino acid that helps to heal the gut. In the early stages of gut healing, taking one teaspoon of glutamine powder (5g) in water last thing at night for two to four weeks helps to heal the gut.

Increase essential fats

Both omega-3 and omega-6 fats are important for gut healing and reducing inflammation. Omega-3 fats are found in oily fish whereas omega-6 fats are found in evening primrose and borage oils. Combination supplements providing omega-3s from fish oil and omega-6 from evening primrose oil and borage oil are the best.

The best vegetarian sources of omega-3 are chia and flax seeds, but these should be ground and soaked, especially during the early stages of recovery.

Consider a shot of aloe vera

Aloe vera juice is very good for digestive health. It contains mucopolysaccharides and acemannan, which help to reduce inflammation in the gut and may accelerate healing. Having a shot of aloe vera juice a day is a good option for digestive health.

Lose weight, exercise and deal with stress

The digestive tract is surrounded by muscles that help move everything along through a snake-like motion called peristalsis. If you take no exercise, lose abdominal muscle strength, gain weight and have a distended gut, this is a recipe for disaster. If you cannot do a sit-up then you have weak abdominal muscles.

Exercises such as yoga and Pilates, and any exercise system that helps to build abdominal muscles, can help digestion. In yoga the exercise called *udiyama* is particularly good (see the next chapter for details).

Following a low-GL diet is one of the most effective ways to lose weight, and the foods included in the diet are naturally high in soluble fibres.

Stress also shuts down proper digestive peristalsis. Therefore, it is important not to eat when you are stressed. Chapter 11 gives you practical solutions for reducing stress when you are about to eat.

Haemorrhoids (piles)

Another consequence of chronic constipation is haemorrhoids. These are swollen blood vessels in and around the anus and rectum that stretch under pressure, much like a varicose vein. The most common reason for the development of haemorrhoids is straining on defecation.

Therefore, the less compacted and the softer the stool, the easier it is to pass. The main symptom of haemorrhoids is anal itching (which can be present in candidiasis infection or in inflammatory bowel disease), which, in turn, can lead to excessive scratching, which further aggravates the condition. Stress can aggravate haemorrhoids.

Although frequent warm baths and anti-inflammatory creams can relieve symptoms, long-term relief is achieved, as for constipation, by dietary changes.

Dietary changes are important but they are not always enough to completely cleanse the intestinal tract. A combination of particular fibres, such as psyllium husks, beet fibre, oat fibre and herbs, which help to loosen up old faecal material, can be beneficial. My favourite is glucomannan fibre. Another helpful treatment is colonic therapy. This is an advanced enema where water is passed into the bowel and, together with abdominal massage, helps to release and remove old faecal material.

Exercise that stimulates the abdominal area can also improve digestion, as do breathing exercises that relax the abdomen. It is a natural reflex of the body to stop digesting in times of stress, so relaxation is important, as you will see in the next chapter.

Summary – Chapter 26

To correct constipation, diverticulitis and haemorrhoids and alleviate discomfort:

- Minimise your intake of meat, dairy, wheat, alcohol and coffee.
- Increase your intake of soluble fibres such as psyllium husks, oat fibre and chia seeds. The best source is glucomannan fibre.
- Re-inoculate the gut with essential fats, beneficial bacteria or digestive enzymes at the start of a meal to maintain a healthy intestinal environment.

- Consider home-made kefir and a daily shot of aloe vera juice.
- Try the mild laxative foods listed on page 282 for one week or opt for powdered fructo-oligosaccharides or chicory root fibre. If you are taking conventional laxatives, ensure adequate hydration.
- Consider weight loss and physical activity, as well as ways to cope with stress.

CHAPTER 27

Abdominal Tension, the Importance of Peristalsis and Gut Yoga

T he digestive system cannot be separated from the rest of the body, nor the body from the mind. Our level of stress and psychological state, therefore, have a lot to do with our digestive health. The digestive system is the basis of our survival, so it represents the instinct for self-preservation. Its physical territory is the abdominal cavity and its centre is the belly.

In the martial-arts tradition the centre of vital energy is located in a point four finger-widths below the belly-button and about 2.5cm in. This is known in different traditions as the *Kath*, *ki* centre, *hara* or *tan-tien*. The abdominal cavity is separated from the thoracic cavity (the lungs, heart and kidneys, contained within the ribcage) by the diaphragm, a dome-shaped muscle. The way we breathe and the action of the diaphragm muscle are critical to our digestive processes. In a relaxed and healthy person the diaphragm muscle is pulled downwards as we inhale, opening up lung space for air to enter; and it is contracted upwards, reducing lung space as we exhale. Therefore, the belly should extend as we inhale, as the diaphragm muscle descends, and it should relax on the out-breath. This is what happens in babies and in animals but, as we get older, many of us lose this natural, deep-breathing ability and instead take very shallow breaths. It is almost as if these two cavities have become disconnected which, in turn, means the digestive organs do not get 'massaged' by the movements of the diaphragm muscle. It also means the muscles of the abdomen may stay in a state of tension, inhibiting the digestive processes.

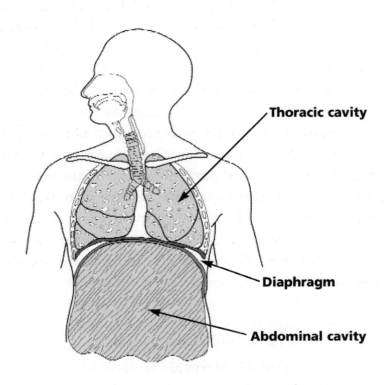

The abdominal and thoracic cavities and
the diaphragm muscle

Although the heart, or thoracic cavity, is said to represent our instinct to relate to others, the belly or abdominal cavity is connected to our instinct for self-preservation, our 'being'. The head or cranial cavity represents our instinct to adapt – how we are in the world. Psychological tensions about doing (coping), relating (belonging) and being (feeling safe) manifest in the body as physical tension. One major area of physical tension is the abdominal muscles. Tension in this area can be seen as a manifestation of the psychological perception of some kind of threat to our existence with thoughts such as 'What if I lose my job?', or 'What if I can't pay the mortgage?', or 'I'll never have enough to feel secure', or 'I don't feel safe' (that is, issues involving our being – food, health, home, money, security, and so on). Psychological tension is stored in the body as physical tension, which has a real impact on digestion, interfering with the normal peristaltic action of the muscles that surround the small and large intestines.

Normally, this peristaltic, snake-like wave of muscle contractions is what keeps everything moving along the digestive tract. If, however, it is suppressed, either by abdominal tension or by constipation and distension of the colon, peristalsis might be effectively blocked or weakened, which leads to an even greater tendency to constipation. Conversely, excessive contraction of the abdominal muscles can result in cramp-like digestive pain and a tendency to diarrhoea.

Relaxing the belly and re-establishing peristalsis

There are several ways to restore proper abdominal muscle tone and peristalsis. These include methods of breathing, abdominal exercises, massage, colonic therapy and muscle-relaxing herbs. All these approaches can be helpful for a wide variety of digestive problems, from abdominal cramping and irritable bowel syndrome (see Chapter 23), to constipation and indigestion. So too can tackling the psychological issues and stresses that lead to abdominal tension.

Breathing exercises

Different schools of yoga and martial arts teach various breathing exercises designed to encourage full, deep breathing, which strengthens and fully utilises the diaphragm muscle. One method I particularly like is called Diakath Breathing™ and is part of an exercise system known as Psychocalisthenics®, authored by Oscar Ichazo. The instructions for Diakath Breathing are given in many of my books, including *The Ten Secrets of 100% Healthy People*.

Abdominal exercises

Conventional exercise focuses on pulling in the belly to look slim and, in men, developing the six-pack look, but it is also important for the abdominal area to be able to relax properly and extend with the breath. While abdominal muscle-strengthening exercises such as sit-ups are good, you also need other kinds of abdominal exercise such as *udiyama*, a classic yoga exercise that helps to stimulate the digestion and massages the organs in the abdominal region.

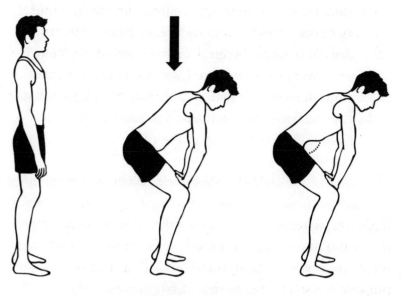

FOOT POSITION: 3 foot-widths
BREATHING: *Inhale,* 3 beats *Exhale,* 3 beats
Hold breath, contract and release muscles, 9 beats
Repeat 3 times.

Udiyama

(NOTE Do not do this exercise if you are pregnant or menstruating.)

1. Bend your knees and place your hands on your thighs just above the knees with your fingers pointing inwards. Your shoulders, arms and hands are relaxed. Your spine and neck are straight. To get the correct 45-degree inclination, bend your knees and tilt your torso and head forward, bringing your hands to rest lightly on your thighs. Your head and spine are in a straight line. Avoid bending over too far. Check the buttock muscles; they should remain relaxed.
2. Exhale sharply, empty your lungs and force the stomach out. Keeping the lungs empty, alternately

contract and relax the abdominal muscles in rapid succession nine times. Make each contraction as deep as possible. Keep the movements of the belly smooth and regular. The correct stance makes the contraction of the *Rectus abdominis* muscle massage the viscera most effectively. You can feel the pull from the pubis bone up to the throat.

This is one of 23 exercises included in a 20-minute routine called Psychocalisthenics. The exercise routine, in its entirety, represents a wonderful way to enliven the body, maintain fitness, strength and suppleness, and improve digestion (see Resources). A complete yoga workout would include such abdominal exercises plus others for rejuvenation and generating energy.

Massage

Although conventional massage rarely delves into releasing tension in the abdominal region, a good massage therapist can encourage the release of abdominal tension. Most of us hold tension in that area, especially when we are under stress; however, care must be taken with such massage in people with inflammatory bowel disease.

Colonic therapy

During a 'colonic', water is passed gently into the colon, and this stimulates the peristaltic muscle action. A good colonic therapist (see Resources) massages the abdominal area during the session in a way that encourages peristaltic muscle action. To re-establish peristaltic muscle action, which can be felt much like a heartbeat, it is best to see a colonic therapist every two or three days until peristalsis is back to normal. This is very helpful for people with a history of constipation, although it would be best to start it after a couple of months of good dietary practices.

Muscle-relaxing herbs

Peppermint is a powerful muscle-relaxing herb. As we have seen, peppermint oil capsules have proven highly effective in people who have abdominal muscle cramping, particularly in irritable bowel syndrome. These, ideally enteric-coated, capsules are swallowed, then released into the upper part of the digestive tract and, if muscle contraction is part of the problem, they can provide significant and relatively immediate relief; however, bear in mind that such muscle contractions can often be the body's way of saying that it is not receiving what it needs in terms of healing foods, so look closely at what you are eating.

Summary – Chapter 27

Some approaches to relieve psychological and associated gastric tension, as well as a variety of digestive problems, include:

- Practising breathing and abdominal exercises.
- Consulting a good colonic or massage therapist.
- Using muscle-relaxing herbs such as peppermint to alleviate abdominal muscle cramping.

CHAPTER 28

Say No to Digestive Cancers

Cancers of the digestive tract are, more often than not, the consequence of long-term neglect of digestive well-being in the form of poor diet, infections and a high intake of digestive irritants. Cancers of the digestive tract itself (mouth, oesophagus, stomach, colon and rectum) are most strongly linked to diet, whereas cancers of the liver and pancreas are somewhat more nebulous in origin. In any event, following the advice for restoring digestive health in Part IV of this book is the best way to minimise your risk.

Mouth, throat and oesophageal cancer

The location of these cancers is strongly suggestive of ingested or inhaled carcinogens. Known risk factors are alcohol, smoking, a lack of fruit and vegetables, and a high intake of maté tea (a hot herbal infusion from South America that is traditionally drunk through a metal straw) or very hot drinks. Alcohol consumption above one drink per day for women or two drinks per day for men increases risk, but the combination of smoking and drinking particularly increases the risk of oesophageal cancer. The most protective nutrients are antioxidants, especially vitamin C, vitamin A and selenium, alongside a diet high in fruit and vegetables and low in alcohol. Don't drink very hot drinks and, needless to say, avoid smoking.

Stomach cancer

Stomach cancer affects 12,000 people a year in the UK. It is very strongly linked to dietary carcinogens, so it is prevented both by avoiding high-risk foods and having a good intake of nutrients, which can disarm carcinogens in food. Known contributory factors are an excess of salt and salted foods; grilled, fried, barbecued or burnt meat; a lack of refrigeration, which increases the risk of pathogens in food; and a low intake of fresh fruit and vegetables.

Stomach cancer starts in the lining of the stomach – which is normally protected from damage by mucus secretions – so it is very likely that digestive irritation is a key trigger. A lack of stomach acid, a lack of nutrients, such as vitamin A (which strengthens the stomach lining), and a high intake of 'irritating' foods such as coffee, alcohol or fried foods are some factors that could lead to irritation. One job of stomach acid is to effectively sterilise the stomach, so a lack of it increases the risk of infection with pathogens such as *Helicobacter pylori* (see Chapter 17 for more on low levels of stomach acid).

A diet high in very salty foods increases the risk of stomach cancer. Stomach cancer levels are very high in Japan where very salty pickled and cured foods, such as kimchee, are popular. Both salt and nitrates used in curing are known risk factors for gastritis. The Japanese suffer more from gastritis, a precursor for stomach cancer, and consequently *Helicobacter pylori*.[97]

Antioxidant nutrients, such as beta-carotene, vitamin C and selenium, help to reduce the risk. Regular consumption of non-starchy vegetables, allium vegetables (such as onions, leeks and garlic), fruits and pulses (beans, peas and lentils, and soya and soya products) is also protective.

Pancreatic cancer and liver cancer

One of the jobs of the pancreas is to produce enzymes to digest foods. This less common type of cancer interferes with digestion, making optimal nutrition difficult. It is often diagnosed after a person starts to experience chronic indigestion and loss of weight. Exactly why it occurs is not known, although risk factors do include a low intake of fruit and vegetables, a low intake of fibre, a high consumption of meat, smoking, and possibly also excessive coffee consumption, although not all studies agree.

The liver is the primary organ of detoxification, and liver cancer is highly indicative of overexposure to, and/or an inability to detoxify, carcinogens. Improving detoxification potential might reduce risk (see Chapter 25). Excess alcohol is the greatest single risk factor, as is the use of certain drugs, including Tamoxifen (the most commonly prescribed drug for breast cancer). Certain types of hepatitis also increase the risk.

All the advice in this book for restoring digestive health is ideal for minimising the chance of developing liver cancer, including avoiding coffee and cigarettes, eating plenty of fruit and vegetables and limiting meat and alcohol. In the case of pancreatic cancer, taking digestive enzymes and specially prepared food, soups and juices might be necessary to help the digestion and absorption of nutrients. Cruciferous vegetables such as broccoli, cauliflower, kale, cabbage and Brussels sprouts help the liver to detoxify.

Colorectal cancer

Bowel (colorectal) cancer is the second most prevalent cancer in the UK – each year more than 30,000 people are diagnosed with the disease, and around 18,000 die of it. Colon cancer is one the fastest-growing cancers, especially in younger adults. A recent US study in the *Journal of the American Medical Association* shows a decline in colorectal cancer in those over the age of 50 but an increase in younger people, and predicts a 50 per cent increase in incidence by 2020, and a doubling by 2030 in people aged 20–34 years old.[98] Colorectal is the third fastest-growing cancer, just behind breast and prostate cancer. To put this into context, in 2013 there were 143,000 diagnoses and 51,000 deaths in the US.

If the cancer is detected in its early stages, there is an 85 per cent chance that it can be cured, but unfortunately many people are diagnosed too late. The correct diet and lifestyle is conservatively estimated to be able to reduce the incidence by 60 per cent.[99]

Although between 5 and 10 per cent of sufferers have a genetic predisposition to bowel cancer, there is no doubt that it is linked to diet and lifestyle. Carcinogens in what we eat, exacerbated by putrefying food (because of poor digestion and constipation) and microorganisms in an unhealthy gut, play a big part. The greatest risk factors are eating a diet high in animal fats and meat (especially grilled, barbecued or burnt) and low in fibre, a history of polyps, smoking, excess alcohol, a lack of exercise, a lack of vegetables, a high calorie intake and prolonged stress.

One of Britain's top bowel experts, Roger Leicester, says, 'Bowel cancer is more likely to develop when people eat a lot of animal fat and there is slow-moving transit of food in the gut.' I have been warning people for years that the combination of carcinogens from burnt animal fat, called HCAs and PAHs, and processed and cured meat which produce carcinogenic nitrosamines, coupled with constipation is a recipe for colorectal cancer. A recent article in the *American Journal of Clinical Nutrition* confirms this link.[100] According to both the World Cancer Research Fund and the American Institute of Cancer, the evidence of an association between red and processed meat and colorectal cancer is convincing. The World Health Organisation classifies processed meats such as bacon, sausages and ham as carcinogens.

A high-fibre diet shortens the time food takes to pass through the digestive tract and thereby reduces carcinogen exposure. In other words, we can minimise our risk of developing colorectal cancer by choosing a diet high in fibre, which helps things move along more quickly, and low in meat, which takes longer to digest. Fibre helps to reduce the 'availability' of carcinogenic compounds. Soluble fibre acts as fuel for the growth of friendly bacteria which, in turn, lower the pH (and therefore raise the acidity) of the colon. Higher acidity is associated with a lower risk of developing colorectal cancer.

One study examined the faecal pH of South Asian vegetarian pre-menopausal women compared with white vegetarian and white omnivorous women to see whether there was any link between this and their intakes of fibre, fat and cholesterol. The research found that there was indeed an association between high-fibre diets and faecal pH. It also showed that such a diet decreased the concentration of bile acids in faeces, a factor which has been linked to a lowered chance of developing colorectal cancer.[101] A high-fat, low-fibre, high-refined-carbohydrate diet also increases the activity of beta-glucuronidase, an enzyme secreted by toxic bacteria, which can generate carcinogens in the colon.[102] The activity of this enzyme can be measured in a stool test such as the Comprehensive Digestive Stool Analysis (see Resources), which a clinical nutritionist can arrange for you.

The protective effect of cruciferous vegetables (such as Brussels sprouts, cabbage, cauliflower and broccoli) against cancers of the digestive tract is well recognised. A double-blind study using Brussels sprouts suggests that the protective mechanism might involve the natural compound glucosi-nolate. In the study, subjects first ate glucosinolate-containing Brussels sprouts for seven days and then glucosinolate-free sprouts for the same period. After the glucosinolate intake, detoxification enzymes in the colon increased by 30 per cent compared with the glucosinolate-free period.[103] It has been suggested that glucosinolate in cruciferous vegetables enhances the detoxifying enzymes that could increase the body's capacity to withstand the burden of daily exposure to toxins and carcinogens. Particularly important nutrients are beta-carotene, vitamin C, folic acid, vitamin D, calcium and selenium. Diet, however, is the major preventative factor. Regular garlic consumption reduces the risk, as does live yoghurt, because it provides beneficial bacteria to improve intestinal health. Supplementing antioxidant nutrients, such as vitamin C, beta-carotene and vitamin E, has been shown to reverse polyps. Although not all polyps lead to colorectal cancer, certain kinds indicate the beginning of a process which, if not reversed, can eventually result in cancerous growths. The presence of polyps, therefore, indicates the need to jump into action with a diet and supplement programme to restore digestive health (see Part IV).

Folic acid and colorectal cancer

There is something else to be aware of, and that is the good and bad sides of folates and folic acid. Folates, the B vitamins found in greens and beans, are strongly associated with a reduced risk of colorectal cancer, probably because they protect the DNA from damage. The trouble with food folates is they are rather unstable, so the supplement industry invented folic acid, a much more stable form. Folic acid has to be converted into the active tetrahydrofolate (THF) form to work, and there is increasing evidence that not everyone is that good at making this conversion in their body. The concern about this is that too much unconverted folic acid in the colon can actually stimulate the growth of pre-existing colorectal cancer cells. Hence, for those at risk – who perhaps don't have a great diet, have a tendency to drink, and are aged over 50 – I don't recommend supplementing above 300mcg of folic acid. Ideally, those people should also test their homocysteine, because it is only those with high homocysteine who might benefit from more folic acid. Fortunately, two stable compounds of active THF have become available, so it is best to choose homocysteine-lowering formulas that use a form of THF instead of folic acid.

Wheat, celiac disease and cancer

As I explained in Chapter 20, the other known risk factor for cancers of the digestive tract is wheat for those who have undiagnosed celiac disease. Gliadin, the main gluten protein in wheat, acts as an intestinal irritant. Oats contain no gliadin and, being high in soluble fibres, help to move everything through.

If you are mindful of these factors and adjust your diet accordingly, colorectal cancer should not be something to worry about.

Summary – Chapter 28

Digestive cancers are preventable. Here are the steps I recommend:

- Increase your intake of soluble fibres, particularly from oats and chia seeds.
- Minimise your intake of processed meat.
- Minimise your intake of fatty, fried, barbecued, grilled and crispy meats, especially red meats.
- Don't drink more than one unit (for women) or two units (for men) of alcohol a day.
- Eat a digestion-friendly diet, as explained in this book.
- Re-inoculate your gut from time to time, or after an infection or excessive drinking, with probiotics or natural yoghurt.
- Eat plenty of antioxidant-rich fruit and, especially, vegetables, particularly cruciferous vegetables.
- Don't add salt to your food, and stay away from very salty foods.
- Smoking, lack of exercise and excessive weight are also risk factors to avoid.

PART IV

RESTORING DIGESTIVE HEALTH

CHAPTER 29

Your Action Plan for Healthy Digestion

The good news for sufferers of digestive discomfort is that you can restore the health of your digestion in weeks – not months. Digestive enzymes take minutes to work – not hours. The epithelial cells that make up the gut wall, maintaining its integrity, take days – not weeks – to be rejuvenated. Probiotics restore gut microbiota in weeks – not months.

Within two weeks you can realistically transform your gut health, providing you are not already in the grips of a gut-related disease. If you are, a month will be a more realistic time frame for digestive transformation. In this chapter, I will guide you towards better digestion, depending on your particular digestive health issue.

14 days to better digestion

The simplest way to transform your gut health in 14 days is to take five simple actions:

1. Follow the Digestion-Friendly Diet in the next
   chapter.
2. Supplement digestive enzymes with each meal.
3. Supplement probiotics twice a day.
4. Take one teaspoon (5g) or three capsules of
   glucomannan with a full glass of water before
   breakfast.
5. Take a basic optimum-nutrition daily supplement
   of vitamins, minerals, plus essential fats (both
   omega-3 and omega-6), plus extra vitamin C (see
   page 325).

In fact, it gets even easier than the above, because there are
supplements that combine digestive enzymes with probiotics,
and some also include glutamine. This perfect trio is taken
one with each meal. When you follow these digestion supplement suggestions, and take a daily shot of super fibres and
follow the Digestion-Friendly Diet, you will reap rewards in
a matter of days.

For optimal health all round, I also recommend everyone
takes the fifth item on the above list: a daily supplement
of an optimum-nutrition multivitamin and mineral, with
extra vitamin C and an essential omega-3 and -6 capsule. I
take these every day. They can also be taken in daily strips
or sachets, taken twice a day. (You can complete the 100%
Health Check online and it will work out your own ideal
personalised supplement programme. See Resources.)

All these supplements, how to find the right ones, and how
to take them, are explained in Chapter 31.

After 14 days, if you are reasonably healthy, you won't
need to keep taking the digestive enzymes or probiotics,
because your good digestive and healthy microbiota will be
established. If there are particular foods that you find hard

to digest, you might find that taking digestive enzymes permanently with meals containing those foods makes all the difference. However, if this simple 14-day digestive tune-up doesn't resolve your issues you need to dig a little deeper.

What's your problem?

The flow chart overleaf will help you find out more and personalise your own plan for restoring digestive health. These are the kinds of tests and treatments a nutritional therapist will employ if you decide that you would like to work with an expert to help you reach the promised land of healthy digestion. (See Resources to find a registered nutritional therapist near you.)

Start at the top of the left-hand column. The worst-case scenario is that you have everything, in which case take all the actions in the dark action boxes, although this is rather unlikely. If you've read the chapters describing each of these health issues, you'll understand why I am making these recommendations. In Chapter 31 each of the specific supplements mentioned is explained so that you'll know what to buy and when to take them.

A more likely scenario is that you have one or two of the problems in the left-hand column; for example, if you experience indigestion, start by following the Digestion-Friendly Diet explained in the next chapter, and take digestive enzymes with each meal. If that doesn't resolve your problem, the next step is to have an IgG food intolerance test (see Resources) and then to avoid the foods you are intolerant to.

If you also, or still have, bad bloating, you could just take a probiotic supplement and see what happens.

*

How to personalise your digestive health recovery programme

Do you have...

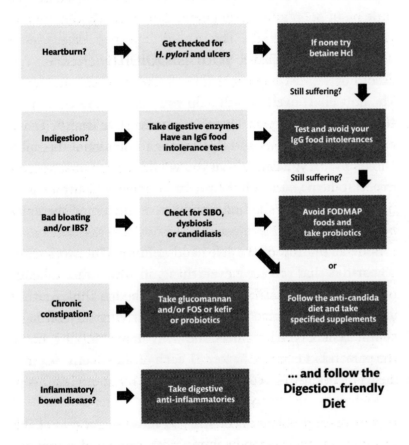

If you actually got worse on my Digestion-Friendly Diet, try eliminating all the FODMAP foods in this diet. These are normal, healthy foods that provide prebiotics that feed your healthy bacteria. The trouble is, if you have SIBO, as we have seen, they may feed unhealthy bacteria too, so you need to avoid these foods until you've restored your good gut health. It's a bit like feeding your flower-bed with nitrogen to boost the flowers. If it's full of weeds, they will grow very well too.

First, you need to do a bit of weeding by restoring a stronger colony of healthy bacteria.

Ideally, in this scenario, you would have gone to a nutritional therapist who has run a digestive stool analysis (you scoop a little bit of poop into a container at home and send it, by registered post, to the lab). This would help them determine if you have SIBO, dysbiosis or candidiasis, and then advise you accordingly. (See Chapters 21–24 for more on these conditions.)

If you have heartburn, there's no harm in taking digestive enzymes and probiotics, and following the Digestion-Friendly Diet as a starting point. This is the 'fall back' position for everyone. But if this doesn't resolve your problem, it is well worth having a medical check for the possibility of *Helicobacter pylori* infection and/or ulcers. Watch out though – many doctors' default position is to give people PPI drugs. (See Chapter 13 for the truth about these drugs and why you are better off exploring the safer natural options in this book first.) If you don't have an ulcer and don't have *H. pylori*, try taking a supplement of betaine hydrochloride (betaine HCl), following the protocol in Chapter 17 for resolving acid reflux, where the dose is gradually increased until you find what works for you.

If your main problem is constipation, and you want a quick result, take one teaspoon (5g), or three capsules, of glucomannan powder with a large glass of water before each meal and stick to the Digestion-Friendly Diet. You might also try probiotics or a daily kefir drink. One of these, plus the Digestion-Friendly Diet, is likely to keep you regular and restore normal peristalsis for effortless elimination. If you are really stuck, there are natural laxative herbs such as senna and cascara, but these override the body's normal peristaltic action and therefore hinder you restoring normal gut contractions. Chapters 26 and 27 explain what to do to help re-establish healthy peristalsis.

Reduce supplements and digestive aids after a month

Within a month, many of these extra supplements will become unnecessary. You don't need to keep taking probiotics, for example, once you've re-established a healthy gut flora. You could top up with the odd probiotic capsule when you've drunk too much alcohol or if you get a return of symptoms.

You will have learnt when you need digestive enzyme supplements, so keep them in reserve.

I take three capsules of glucomannan powder once a day, but not every day – I take them especially on those days when my breakfast isn't high in soluble fibres.

If you previously suffered from heartburn and indigestion, but got significant relief from supplementing betaine HCl, you might want to explore the lowest dose that gives you relief. If you are older, you might find that you need to keep taking this because your body is just not able to make enough to optimise digestion and therefore needs ongoing support. Be sure to also check your homocysteine level and supplement B vitamins, especially B_{12}, accordingly, because the older you get the more you are likely to need them.

The next chapter explains what to eat and drink for a healthy digestive system.

Summary – Chapter 29

If you feel that you can benefit from improving your digestive system I recommend that you:

- Follow the five essential steps to transform your gut health in 14 days on page 308.
- Supplement a combination formula of digestive enzymes, probiotics and glutamine with each meal. Supplementation of these is not essential once your intestinal environment has been restored.
- Avoid the foods you react to (and, if necessary, the FODMAP foods) and follow the recommended Digestion-Friendly Diet.
- Consider a digestive stool analysis to determine if you have SIBO, dysbiosis or candidiasis or other microbial infections.
- Follow my guidelines to alleviate constipation in Chapter 27. For quick results, take 5g of glucomannan powder with a large glass of water before each meal when needed.
- For ongoing digestive support, you may encounter relief from supplementing betaine HCl. If you are older, ensure frequent monitoring of homocysteine levels and appropriate B_{12} supplementation if you are on antacid PPI drugs.

CHAPTER 30

The Digestion-Friendly Diet

Throughout the centuries, health experts have extolled the value of spring-cleaning the body. In much the same way as you need a holiday from work, your body needs a break from detoxifying, which is a natural process in your body that goes on continually. One of the traditional methods of purifying the body is through fasting. Many people report feeling so much more vital after fasting, and this is testimony to the fact that making energy is as much a result of improving the body's ability to detoxify as it is about eating the correct foods.

Not everybody feels better for fasting, however, or not always immediately. A common occurrence is the so-called 'healing crisis' when a person feels worse for a few days and then feels better. What we are learning about detoxification processes suggests that some people might be experiencing a health crisis rather than a healing crisis. Once the body starts to liberate and eliminate toxic material, if the liver isn't up to the job, symptoms of detox overload can result. Hence, modern detox regimes tend to use modified fasts, in which the person is given a low-toxin diet, plus plenty of the key nutrients needed to speed up the body's ability to detoxify.

Doing this once a year, for a couple of weeks, can make a major difference to your energy levels. I favour this approach and have had nothing but great feedback on my 9-Day Liver Detox Diet. This detox diet eliminates wheat, milk, sugar, alcohol, caffeine and damaged, burnt fats for nine days, and advocates eating highly nutritious foods that are plentiful in natural antioxidants and are anti-inflammatory. The diet is also enhanced through taking specific supplements.

My Digestion-Friendly Diet is based on similar principles, but is focused specifically on gut health rather than liver function. Of course, you can keep doing it if you want to. Many people feel so good eating this way it becomes their norm.

What our research told us about a diet for a healthy digestion

In this chapter I want to establish the basics of a Digestion-Friendly Diet. A good place to start is our research on over 100,000 people who have taken the 100% Health Check questionnaire. When we analysed the diets of the first 55,570 people, we could see what the difference was in the diets of those with the best and worst digestive health. On the foll-lowing page you'll find the results in order of best and worst.

Of all the body systems we investigated, digestion was the only health factor for which a form of sugar was *not* the most impactful food group. Red meat consumption more than eight times per week increased the likelihood of very poor digestive health by two-thirds, with salt- and sugar-based snacks also showing strong negative associations. The likelihood of very poor digestive health was over one and a half times greater in those who consumed more than seven portions of red meat per week than those who consumed less or none; by contrast,

the high consumption of nuts and seeds reduced the likelihood of very poor digestive health by a third, significantly the
most positively associated food.

The best foods for digestive health	The worst foods for digestive health
Nuts and seeds	Red meat
Fresh fruit	Sugar-based snacks
Oily fish	Salt
Vegetables/salad	Added sugar
Water	Wheat
	Dairy
	Refined foods
	Tea/coffee/cola
	Processed meals

This might not sit well with the Paleo, Atkins and Banting
diet supporters (who eat meat regularly), but this is what we
found in this rather large survey. There are also those who
shun pulses (lentils, beans and chickpeas) for a number of
reasons. Firstly, on the grounds that our Palaeolithic ancestors
wouldn't have eaten them; secondly, that they contain lectins,
which the body's immune system fights against; and thirdly
that they are hard to digest. All 'seed' foods are hard to digest,
however, because the plant wants the animal to eat it but not
to digest it, and then to deposit it in a nice manure-rich starter
kit some distance away from the original tree or bush. On the
other hand, it is exactly these 'seed' foods that contain the most
nutrients. Mankind has learnt how to crack open the nut, grind
the seed, cook, sprout or ferment the bean to both maximise
their nutrient absorption and render them easier to digest. Also,
more than half the population of the world – the healthier half,

from India, China, Japan, Thailand and Malaysia – who have among the lowest cancer, diabetes and heart disease rates in the world, eat pulses as staple foods. An exception to this is the high rate of stomach cancer in Japan, most strongly linked to salted and cured foods (see page 297). In our survey, salt was strongly linked to digestive problems.

As our survey showed, those with the healthiest diges-tion ate the most nuts and seeds. (Unfortunately our survey couldn't separate out beans.) Therefore, unless you are specif-ically intolerant to these foods or unable to digest them (even when having the most suitable digestive-enzyme support), or if you are producing too much gas, and have bloating and dis-comfort, as some with IBS do, these are not 'bad' foods. They are positively good for you, unless you have compromised digestion and dysbiosis, in which case they might need to be limited until you restore your digestive health.

Your quick-look guide to foods

Looked at from a physiological point of view, a Digestion-Friendly Diet should *include* foods and drinks that are:

- High in soluble fibres that encourage healthy elimination.
- High in prebiotics that encourage a healthy microbiota.
- Fermented, high in probiotics or, at least, producing lactic acid.
- Nutritious and easy to digest.
- High in antioxidants and anti-inflammatory nutrients.

A Digestion-Friendly Diet should *exclude* foods and drinks that:

- Increase gut permeability and inflame the gut.
- Kill healthy bacteria and encourage unhealthy microbiota.
- Slow down elimination.

On that basis, these are the foods that make up a Digestion-Friendly Diet:

Eat:
All vegetables, including *onions* and *garlic* – organic if possible
Apples and pears, unripe bananas
Avocados, asparagus, *artichokes*
Beans, peas, chickpeas and *lentils* (soaked, well cooked or fermented)
Berries, *cherries, plums*
Brown rice
Dairy-free yoghurt cultured with *Lactobacillus* and bifidobacteria
Eggs, free-range, organic
Fish, especially oily fish (poached, steamed or baked)
Ginger, turmeric, oregano, mint
Kamut khorasan wheat, pasta and bulgar (unless you have celiac disease)
Kefir
Oatcakes
Oat milk
Oats – raw or cooked
Quinoa
Raw nuts including *cashew nuts, pistachio nuts,* almonds and seeds, especially chia seeds
Sauerkraut
Spouted seeds and grains

Sugar-free yoghurt cultured with *Lactobacillus* and
  bifidobacteria (unless dairy intolerant)
Tofu, tempeh, hummus
Whole sweetcorn, whole maize flour (polenta/
  cornmeal), millet
Xylitol, *inulin*, as sweeteners
Water
Green tea and peppermint (maximum 3 a day)
Herb teas such as rooibos (red bush), moringa with
  ginger
Montmorency *cherry concentrate* (CherryActive), diluted

Limit:

Alcohol (choose organic wines, champagne method,
  spirits)
Chilli (cayenne and paprika are better)
Coffee and strong tea (maximum 1 a day)
Dairy products (unless intolerant)
Fruit juice
Lean organic red meat
Lean organic white meat
Ripe bananas, grapes, dates, raisins, dried fruit (except
  blueberries and prunes)
Rye, barley, durum wheat pasta
Unheated honey, organic agave syrup

Avoid:

Added salt, MSG and other chemical additives
Deep-fried food
Food additives and preservatives
French fries
High-yeast alcohols (beers, cheap wine)
Modern wheat

Processed meats
Fatty red meat
Sugar and artificial sweeteners
Yeasted breads

NOTE Those foods shown in italics are best avoided for the first week if you suffer from IBS or SIBO, as explained in Chapter 23.

Digestion-friendly recipes

What do you actually eat to put all these digestion-friendly nutrition principles into practice? Part V provides digestion-friendly breakfasts, lunches, dinners and snacks, all designed to keep your digestive system healthy.

If you have particular food intolerances or need to be following a low-FODMAP diet as part of your digestion-recovery strategy, some of the recipes using beans and lentils might not work for you in the short term; however, once your digestion is working, helped by a period of time on enzymes and probiotics, these foods, which are high in nutrients and prebiotics, will help to keep you healthy.

I have selected recipes, created by my co-author and kitchen wizard Fiona McDonald Joyce, from our three favourite books, *The 9-Day Liver Detox Diet*, *The Ten Secrets of 100% Health Cookbook* and *Delicious, Healthy, Sugar-Free*. These books have many more recipes to help you expand your repertoire.

The recipes are based on fresh, healthy ingredients that are free from digestive irritants and naturally rich in nutrients that aid digestion. This will get you started and give you plenty of ideas for putting the Digestion-Friendly Diet into practice. A typical day's menu might look like this, including a FODMAP-friendly day:

Sample menus

Day 1:

Breakfast Cinnamon Fruit Porridge (page 336)
Lunch Curried Pumpkin Soup (page 353)
Dinner Thai Chicken and Cashew Nut Stir-Fry (page 378)
Snack/s Apple, a handful walnuts/corn on the cob (page 381)

Day 2:

Breakfast Chia Pancakes with Pear Compote (page 340)
Lunch Butternut Squash and Tenderstem Broccoli Salad (page 349)
Dinner Salmon with Puy Lentils (page 365)
Snack/s Blueberry Yoghurt Sundae (page 384)/2–3 rough oatcakes with nut butter

Day 3:

Breakfast: Hot-Smoked Trout with Scrambled Eggs and Watercress (page 341)
Lunch Superfood Salad of Quinoa with Roasted Veg (page 347)
Dinner Baked Sweet Potatoes with Borlotti Stew (page 356)
Snack/s Crudités with Hummus (page 384)/pear, a handful almonds

FODMAP-friendly sample day:

Breakfast Kippers with Wilted Spinach (page 342)
Lunch Butternut Squash and Tenderstem Broccoli Salad (page 349)

Dinner Moroccan-Style Chicken (omit the onions) (page 376)
Snack/s FODMAP-friendly fruit, such as banana, grapes, melon, orange and berries (see the full list on page 243)/corn on the cob (page 381)

Summary – Chapter 30

An optimal action plan for healthy digestion should aim to cover the following:

* Incorporate modern detox regimes such as my 9-Day Liver Detox Diet, perhaps following this once a year, and my Digestion-Friendly Diet recommendations into your daily regime.
* Adhere to the dos and don'ts of my Digestion-Friendly Diet and adopt the associated dietary practices listed on pages 317–320. The italicised 'harmful' foods should be avoided for one week if your digestive system is sensitive to them.
* Have a look at the digestion-friendly recipes in my three favourite books *The 9-Day Liver Detox Diet, The Ten Secrets of 100% Health Cookbook* and *Delicious, Healthy, Sugar-Free.*

CHAPTER 31

Digestive Supplements

Taken on a regular basis, nutritional supplements composed of vitamins, minerals, essential fats, phospholipids and antioxidants make a big difference to your digestive and overall health. This is because every step of the digestive process, from digestion to detoxification, depends on a whole host of nutrients that are often deficient in our modern diet and almost impossible to obtain at optimal levels from diet alone. These are the cornerstones of a daily supplement programme and will consist of:

- A multivitamin and mineral
- Extra vitamin C
- Essential omega-3 and -6 oils
- Extra antioxidants and phospholipids (optional)

I recommend these to everyone, and I take them myself. These are the basic ingredients of an optimum-nutrition-style daily supplement regime.

Then there are supplements to take either to restore gut health or to deal with your particular area of vulnerability. These include:

- Super-soluble fibres to aid elimination – glucomannan, PGX, psyllium, chia seeds
- Digestive enzymes – protease, amylase, lipase, lactase, glucoamylase, alpha-galactosidase
- Digestive aids – betaine HCl, zinc, lecithin
- Probiotics – *Lactobacillus* and bifidobacteria strains
- Probiotic and prebiotic aids – FOS, inulin, *Saccharomyces boulardii*, kefir
- Gut-wall healers – glutamine and butyric acid, vitamins A and D, zinc
- Liver detox support – glutamine, glutathione, lipoic acid and other antioxidants, slippery elm, silymarin (milk thistle)
- Anti-microbials – caprylic acid, artemisia, oregano oil, olive leaf, berberine (or goldenseal), grapefruit seed extract and garlic
- Anti-spasmodics – peppermint oil, magnesium
- Anti-inflammatories – EPA-rich omega-3, turmeric, quercetin, MSM, bromelain, ginger, aloe vera
- Laxatives – senna, cascara, magnesium, FOS, inulin, xylitol and super-soluble fibres

You do not need to take the above all the time but might call on them to restore digestive health or when things go wrong. I will recommend some of these for short-term use in your digestive health recovery programme, depending on your unique situation. Should you see a nutritional therapist, these are the kinds of supplements that he or she is likely to recommend.

To help you find your way through the maze of natural digestive remedies, to understand what they do and to help you choose the best ones, here is a summary of the key ingredients and the doses you are looking for.

Vitamin and mineral supplements

Multivitamin–mineral The basis of any supplement programme is a good high-strength multivitamin–mineral.
This will contain basic levels of vitamins A, B, C, D and E
plus minerals such as calcium, magnesium, iron, zinc, man-
ganese, chromium and selenium. These nutrients support
digestion, thus maintaining a healthy digestive tract and
liver detoxification. It is vital to have enough vitamin A in
the form of retinol or retinyl (5,000iu/1,500mcg), vitamin
D (600iu/15mcg), zinc (10mg) and magnesium (150mg), as
these all support digestive health. Also, you want to have
enough vitamin B_{12}, especially later in life – 10mcg is a good
basic level. Since water-soluble vitamins are in and out of the
body within six hours, it is best to take a multi twice a day.

Vitamin C is never high enough in a multivitamin because
there's no room for it. You need at least 500–2,000mg a day.
Ascorbic acid works fine, but some people with digestive
problems have a low tolerance for it. If so, try a more alkaline
form of vitamin C, ascorbate, but bear in mind that this must
be attached to a mineral, most often calcium, magnesium,
sodium or potassium ascorbate. If you take high doses – for
example, for fighting a viral infection – you'll be getting a lot
of these minerals. Magnesium relaxes the gut at high doses,
so you might experience a laxative effect (as you would with
milk of magnesia).

Essential omegas include both omega-3 and omega-6.
You need both, but most of us are more likely to be lacking omega-3. The most potent omega-3 for calming down
inflammation is called EPA. DPA also converts to EPA. You

want to be supplementing at least 350mg of these a day, and 1,000–2,000mg for dealing with inflammation.

Antioxidants are vital for protecting against oxidant damage to the digestive tract and liver detoxification. In addition to vitamins A, C and E, and the antioxidant minerals zinc and selenium, which might already be in your multi, good antioxidant supplements should also provide glutathione or NAC (its precursor) and lipoic acid. The older you are, the more you will need.

Phospholipids are semi-essential nutrients, meaning that you can make them but you also need to eat them – fish and eggs being the richest food sources. Lecithin is also a good source. These are optional and good for brain function as well as the gut.

I take a daily pack that provides all these, without fail, every day.

Probiotics

It is not necessary to take probiotic supplements every day, although some health experts recommend it. It is not harmful to do so. They are the best way to re-inoculate the digestive tract with beneficial bacteria after an infection or as part of a strategy for restoring digestive health. There are many different strains of health-promoting bacteria (see Chapter 7), and perhaps there are more to come, as this is a very fertile area of ongoing research. But the two main families are *Lactobacillus* and bifidobacteria. Different blends contain different strains of these. Unless you know exactly what you are going for, it is usually better to buy a blend that includes a number of strains. Whichever you take, make sure that these are present in effective quantities, such as 1 billion or more viable organisms per capsule or serving. Some supplements also contain fructo-oligosaccharides (FOS), which help the bacteria to multiply once they are inside you.

Digestive enzymes

These include a wide variety of enzymes from both animal and plant sources. Look for a supplement that contains lipase (for digesting fat), protease (for digesting protein), amylase (for digesting carbohydrate), amyloglucosidase (for digesting glucosides in certain vegetables), alpha-galactosidase (for digesting beans and pulses) and possibly lactase (for digesting milk sugar), invertase (for digesting sugar) and cellulase (for digesting cellulose). The dose is difficult to specify because they are all measured in different kinds of units of measurement for each enzyme. As a very basic rule of thumb you're probably going to need 20mg or more to make a difference to your digestion.

Papain, from papaya, digests protein; as does bromelain from pineapple. There are also animal-based products such as pancreatin which provide combinations of digestive enzymes.

Digestive aids

If you are lacking stomach acid, you can supplement betaine hydrochloride (betaine HCl), starting at around 300mg a day, with meals. Some people need much more (see Chapter 17). Do not take this if you have an ulcer. Zinc is also needed to make stomach acid, so make sure you are supplementing enough (10–20mg). To further help fat digestion, supplement lecithin, either as granules or capsules.

Probiotic and prebiotic aids

These are FOS, inulin, *Saccharomyces boulardii* and kefir.

Gut-wall healers

A number of supplements exist to help intestinal rebuilding and repair. The key nutrients are vitamin A and zinc, although you also need enough vitamin D. How much you need depends on your blood level, as it stores in the body. A good therapeutic dose of vitamin D for a month is 50mcg/2,000iu. Certain forms of zinc can be irritating to the digestive tract in large amounts. I recommend zinc citrate, ascorbate or amino acid chelate. Glutamine is direct fuel for the intestinal mucosa and a great gut healer. You need 5–10g a day, best taken last thing at night. Supplements are very expensive, but you can buy this amino acid as a powder. It is tasteless and best stirred into cold water – heat destroys it and so does stomach acid, so take it on an empty stomach. Butyric acid, a non-essential fat normally made by intestinal bacteria, also acts as fuel for the intestinal mucosa. You need around 500mg or more a day.

Anti-microbials

There are many remedies specifically designed to give unfavourable microorganisms a hard time. These vary depending on the infection and might include caprylic acid, grapefruit seed extract, artemisia, goldenseal, olive leaf extract, garlic, and many others (see Chapter 21). Consult a nutritional therapist to determine the best dosage levels for your particular digestive problem. These are not nutrients and some will have a negative effect on good bacteria, so they are not meant to be taken every day, just in order to restore digestive health; for example, if you have SIBO or candidiasis.

Anti-inflammatories

These are natural substances that calm down an inflamed gut. Probiotics should be included here because they help too, as does glutamine by restoring gut integrity. EPA-rich omega-3 fish oils are key, followed by highly absorbable forms of curcumin from turmeric, quercetin, MSM, bromelain, ginger and aloe vera. The dosage is the key – you want about 1,000mg of EPA for an anti-inflammatory effect and around the same for both turmeric extract and quercetin, although the turmeric dose depends very much on the form; some are highly bio-available, so you don't need as much; follow the directions on the pack. A daily shot of aloe vera juice and a strong ginger tea helps to calm down a belly on fire. I make ginger juice and freeze it in an ice cube tray, melting a lump of ginger into teas or having a ginger cube in cold drinks.

Anti-spasmodics

Peppermint oil capsules are available as an anti-spasmodic, which means they help to calm down muscular contractions in the digestive tract. Make sure you use an enteric-coated capsule to prevent it breaking down in the stomach so that it can act effectively in the small intestine. The dose that has proven effective is 0.2ml three times a day.

Laxatives

For the immediate relief of constipation, herbal remedies containing either senna or cascara are available. These are mild irritants and are best used only in the short term. Another is milk of magnesia or high-dose magnesium, above 1,000mg. It draws water into stools and thus acts as a laxative. A less drastic way to solve such a problem is to supplement fructo-oligosaccharides (FOS), inulin or xylitol, which increase the transit time by maintaining a higher moisture level in the digestive tract. You need about 5g a day to achieve this. FOS or inulin are better than xylitol, as they are prebiotics; however, bear in mind that if you have SIBO and an excess of unhealthy gut bacteria, these prebiotics will feed them too. If these produce excessive wind and bloating, they are not for you. For many people, increasing super-soluble fibres is sufficient.

Liver-detox support

Some supplements focus specifically on improving the body's ability to detoxify (see Chapter 25). The nutrients needed to support Phase 1 of detoxification are vitamins B_2, B_3, B_6, B_{12}, folic acid, glutathione, branched-chain amino acids, flavonoids and phospholipids, plus a good supply of antioxidant nutrients to disarm dangerous intermediary oxidants created during this stage. Phase 2 of detoxification can be triggered by a specific list of nutrients, including the amino acids glycine, taurine, glutamine and arginine. Cysteine, N-acetyl cysteine and methionine are also precursors for these nutrients (that is, the body can convert these into the others). Combinations of these nutrients are available, together with detoxifying herbs such as milk thistle (which contains silymarin).

Summary – Chapter 31

If you are considering following a daily supplementation programme to support your digestive and detoxification processes, I recommend the following:

- Daily supplementation of a multivitamin and mineral, extra vitamin C, essential omega-3 and -6 oils, extra antioxidants and phospholipids in combination.
- An exhaustive list of the most suitable agents to restore gut integrity and health, whether it's antimicrobial remedies, anti-inflammatory or anti-spasmodic agents, laxatives, prebiotics and probiotics, is provided on page 324.
- Consider various recommended digestive aids to stimulate stomach acid production.
- Include nutrients, amino acids and detoxifying herbs that are known to support the liver's detoxification potential.
- Supplement gut-wall healers such as zinc in the forms of citrate, ascorbate or amino acid chelate at 50mcg per day for one month. Alternatively, 5–10g of glutamine before sleep is also suitable.

PART V

GUTSTRONOMY – RECIPES FOR HEALTHY DIGESTION

CHAPTER 32

Gut-Friendly Breakfasts

B reakfast is the most important meal of the day, and here are a few digestion-friendly recipes to get you off to a good start.

NOTE **ⓕ** = FODMAP friendly

Superfood Muesli

This thick, soaked muesli is delicious and particularly nutritious, as all the ingredients are raw, maximising the vitamin, enzyme and antioxidant content.

Serves 1
40g whole rolled porridge oats
1 tbsp ground almonds or desiccated coconut
1 tbsp Essential Seed Mix
    (see page 337)
½ small apple, grated
1 tbsp berries, such as raspberries or blueberries
½ tsp ground cinnamon, or to taste
    (optional)

Put all the ingredients in a bowl and cover with double the volume of boiling water. Stir and leave to thicken for a couple of minutes until the oats have soaked up the water and become soft and plump.

Cinnamon Fruit Porridge

Oats are full of soluble fibre for healthy digestion. They release their energy slowly, keeping you full for longer. Cinnamon not only adds a wonderfully warming flavour but it is also a valuable nutrient, helping the body to regulate blood-sugar levels.
Ⓕ if you use FODMAP-friendly fruit (see page 241).

Serves 1
40g whole rolled porridge oats
½–1 tsp ground cinnamon, or to taste
1 tbsp Essential Seed Mix (see opposite)
fresh fruit, chopped, grated, or berries left whole

1. Put the oats in a pan over a medium heat and cover with water. Bring to the boil, then simmer gently, stirring frequently, until the porridge thickens and the oats soften.
2. Stir the cinnamon, seed mix and fruit into the porridge, or simply scatter on top of the porridge in a bowl.

Berry Breakfast Smoothie

If you don't have the time or inclination for breakfast, then go for a smoothie. You can drink it on the run and it is packed with nutrients. Try thickening the smoothie with live, natural yoghurt to add extra protein and beneficial probiotic bacteria.

Serves 1
1 small banana, or ½ medium one, not too ripe
2 tsp Essential Seed Mix (see below)
150g blueberries or other berries
juice of ½ lemon
enough unsweetened rice milk, or almond or water, to give
    an easy-to-drink consistency (or leave thick and eat with
    a spoon)

Put all the ingredients in a blender or food processor and blend until smooth.

Essential Seed Mix

1. Half-fill a glass jar that has a sealing lid with a mixture of chia and flax seeds. Fill the remaining half with a mixture of sesame, pumpkin and sunflower seeds. Keep the jar sealed and in the fridge to minimise damage from heat, light and oxygen.
2. Put a handful of the seed mix in a coffee or seed grinder. Grind up and use as indicated in the relevant recipe – or simply sprinkle over your cereal. To save time, you could grind up to one week's worth of seeds, but ensure that you store them away from heat, light and air.

Oat Crunch Yoghurt Pots

Pear and cinnamon are perfect flavour partners and make a great breakfast combo. The protein from the nuts and yoghurt is digested more slowly than carbohydrate, ensuring a steady release of energy.

Serves 4

4 pears, cored and roughly chopped

1 tsp ground cinnamon, or to taste

1 tbsp coconut oil or mild olive oil

2 tbsp xylitol or coconut palm sugar

50g whole oat flakes

1 tbsp flaked almonds

1 tbsp ground chia seeds

1 tbsp roughly chopped macadamia nuts, hazelnuts or any
other raw, unsalted nut

1 tbsp pumpkin seeds

400g live natural yoghurt

1. Put the pears and a dash of water in a pan over a high heat, cover and bring to the boil, then reduce the heat and simmer for 3–5 minutes or until fairly soft. Add a little cinnamon to taste. Set aside to cool.
2. Gently heat the oil in a frying pan over a medium heat, then add the xylitol, oats, nuts and seeds, and stir for a couple of minutes or so to allow the oats to toast slightly. Set aside to cool.
3. Put the stewed pears in small serving bowls, cover with the yoghurt and top with the granola.

Raw Chocolate and Goji Granola

This chewy, chocolatey granola might seem far too decadent for breakfast, but in fact it's a cunningly disguised healthy option. It is packed with seeds, while the cacao powder adds a rich, chocolate flavour but none of the added fat and sugar of processed chocolate. It is also a good source of magnesium – nature's relaxant mineral.

Serves 4
3 tbsp coconut oil or mild olive oil
150g whole oat flakes
3 tbsp tahini
3 tbsp pumpkin seeds
3 tbsp sunflower seeds
3 tbsp sesame seeds
3 tbsp ground chia seeds
3 tbsp desiccated coconut
3 tbsp goji berries
3 tbsp xylitol or coconut palm sugar, or to taste
1 tsp ground cinnamon, or to taste
1 tsp ground ginger, or to taste
4 tbsp raw cacao powder, or to taste

1. Gently heat the oil in a frying pan over a medium heat. Add the oat flakes and stir to coat them with the oil. Then mix in the tahini as best you can, spreading it around the oats fairly evenly.
2. Turn off the heat and stir in the remaining ingredients. Taste and adjust the flavour by adding more xylitol, cinnamon, ginger or cacao, if necessary.

Porridge with Almonds and Goji Berries

Try to buy organic or unsulphured dried fruit in order to avoid the use of the preservative sulphur dioxide, a potential allergen. If you do not have goji berries, try chopped dried apricots instead. If you wish to sweeten the recipe, use a little xylitol.

Serves 1
4 tbsp porridge oats
water or milk/non-dairy milk, or a 50:50 blend

2 tsp–1 tbsp goji berries, to taste

1 tbsp flaked almonds

1. Put the oats in a small pan. Add double the volume of water, milk or a blend of both. Bring to the boil then reduce the heat to a gentle simmer and allow to bubble and thicken for a few minutes, until the oats have swollen.
2. Pour into a bowl, then sprinkle with goji berries and almonds before serving.

Chia Pancakes with Pear Compote

These little pancakes are made with ground oats and chia seeds rather than white flour. The texture is a little coarser, but they are just as moreish and much, much better for you. This recipe makes enough for four people, but the pancakes keep well for a couple of days in the fridge or can be frozen.

Serves 4 (makes 8 pancakes)

45g oats

45g ground chia seeds

35g xylitol or coconut palm sugar

1 organic or free-range egg

225ml milk or non-dairy milk

virgin rapeseed oil, for frying

For the pear compote:

2 large pears, cored and diced

1 tsp ground mixed spice or cinnamon, or to taste

xylitol or coconut palm sugar, to taste (optional)

1. To make the compote, put the pears in a small pan over a medium heat with a tiny dash of water

and the spice. Bring to a simmer, then cover and leave to cook for 5 minutes or until just softened. Taste and add more spice if you like. Sweeten the mixture with the xylitol if you feel it needs it. Set aside, with the lid on, while you make the pancakes.

2. Put the oats in a food processor and add the chia, then grind until as fine as flour. If your food processor leaves the mixture coarse, try a hand blender to achieve a smoother finish.

3. Mix the xylitol into the flour.

4. Whisk the egg and milk together in a bowl and stir into the flour mixture to form a smooth batter. The chia absorbs liquid, so it will thicken more than a standard pancake batter.

5. Heat 1–2 tbsp oil in a large frying pan over a medium-high heat, then spoon in tablespoonfuls of the batter, spreading each out into a rough circle and taking care not to let them touch. Do this in batches and cook each pancake for 1–2 minutes per side, or until golden and firmed up before turning. Press down in the pan to flatten them and help them cook. Put the pancakes onto a warmed plate as they cook, and cover with a tea towel to keep warm. Serve with the compote.

Hot-Smoked Trout with Scrambled Eggs and Watercress

This makes an excellent weekend breakfast for when you have a bit more time to treat yourself. It tastes particularly good served on toasted pumpernickel or sourdough rye bread.

Serves 1
a knob of butter or coconut oil
2 organic or free-range eggs
1 hot-smoked trout fillet
small handful watercress, roughly chopped
freshly ground black pepper
lemon wedge, to serve

1. Melt the butter in a small pan over a gentle heat and crack the eggs into the pan and stir with a wooden spoon to mix.
2. Slowly stir the eggs with a wooden spoon, scraping along the base of the pan as they cook to help stop them sticking. Remove from the heat as soon as the eggs are almost set but still a little runny/moist, as they will carry on cooking in the pan.
3. Spoon the eggs on to a plate, then put the trout fillet on top, sprinkle with black pepper, then scatter the watercress over the top. Serve immediately with a lemon wedge on the side.

Kippers with Wilted Spinach

'Proper' kippers are well worth hunting out from the fishmonger and paying a little extra for. As an oily fish, they provide omega-3 essential fats as well as protein. Omega-3 fats help to reduce gut inflammation, and oily fish provides plenty of other essential vitamins such as B_{12}, phospholipids and vitamin D.

Serves 1
1 undyed, naturally smoked kipper, filleted
a handful of baby leaf spinach

a knob of butter or a drizzle of extra virgin olive oil
(optional)
freshly ground black pepper
lemon wedge, to serve

1. Grill the kipper for 5 minutes or until heated
   through.
2. Meanwhile, put the spinach in a small pan over a
   medium heat and let it wilt for a minute or so. Add
   the butter, if you like.
3. Serve the kipper with the spinach and sprinkle
   with plenty of black pepper. Serve with a lemon
   wedge on the side.

Salmon and Asparagus Omelette

This dish ticks a lot of boxes, with the oily fish providing
omega-3, the egg providing a hefty dose of B vitamins and the
green vegetables adding fibre and vitamins.

Serves 1
50g fine asparagus spears, trimmed
a knob of butter or coconut oil
3 organic or free-range eggs, beaten
1 heaped tbsp diced smoked salmon, or more if you like
freshly ground black pepper
lemon wedge, to serve

1. Steam the asparagus in a steamer insert in a large
   pan containing boiling water for about 5 minutes
   or until al dente – take care to take it off the heat
   as soon as it is cooked. While this is cooking, make
   the omelette.

2. Heat a small frying pan over a medium heat, add the butter and move it about the pan to coat the base and sides, then pour in the eggs. As the omelette starts to set, repeatedly run the back of a fork across the base of the pan to lift up some of the mixture and let the uncooked egg spill underneath and cook.

3. When the base has coloured and set, put the asparagus over half the omelette and top with the smoked salmon. Sprinkle with black pepper, then carefully fold in half and leave for 30 seconds or so to cook the middle before easing it out of the pan and onto a plate. Serve immediately, with a lemon wedge on the side.

CHAPTER 33

Gut-Friendly Main Meals

I n this chapter you will find some recipes for lunches and dinners, with vegan and vegetarian options, also including fish dishes and a few with white meat. There's enough for anyone to be able to choose from. The recipes are also low GL, which means you won't be feeding your gut bacteria with sugar, but you will be taking in a healthy amount of soluble fibres, which also lower the glycemic load of a meal.

NOTE ❶ = FODMAP friendly

Lunches

Superboost Sesame Salad

The strong flavours of toasted sesame oil and lemon juice add flavour to this easy-to-make salad without adding any salt or spices. Serve with a leafy salad, if you like. You can double the quantities if you would like a more substantial meal.

Serves 2

400g can chickpeas, rinsed and drained

2 celery sticks, finely chopped

6 pieces marinated artichoke heart from a jar, roughly chopped

6 spring onions, finely chopped

1 tbsp sesame seeds (untoasted)

1 tsp toasted sesame oil, or to taste

juice of ½ a lemon

Mix all the ingredients together and serve.

Cleansing Bean and Artichoke Salad

This dish is surprisingly filling and full-flavoured, and is equally good served hot or cold. It is packed with digestion-boosting fibre, including inulin in the artichokes, which encourages beneficial probiotic bacteria to flourish in the gut.

Serves 2

1 tbsp coconut oil or 2 tbsp mild olive oil

2 garlic cloves, crushed

1 red onion, finely diced

250g cherry tomatoes, chopped

2 tbsp tomato purée

400g can mixed beans, rinsed and drained

6 marinated artichoke heart halves from a jar, roughly chopped

2 tbsp pitted black olives, roughly chopped (optional)

a handful of fresh basil leaves, torn or Super Greens Mix (see
   opposite)

1. Heat the oil in a frying pan over a medium heat and cook the garlic and onion for 3 minutes or until translucent.

2. Add the tomatoes and cook for 2 minutes or until they disintegrate.

3. Stir in the tomato purée, beans, artichoke hearts and olives, if using, then reduce the heat and simmer for 5 minutes or until thick and rich – you can add a splash of water to loosen it if the sauce dries up. Add the basil or Super Greens Mix just before serving.

Super Greens Mix

This pesto-style blend of dark green leaves and herbs is a brilliant way to increase your intake of these healthy vegetables without having to wade through buckets of salad. Serves 1. Put a good handful of each of the following into a mini-blender or food processor: watercress, baby spinach leaves, basil leaves and parsley leaves. Add 1 tbsp extra virgin olive oil or an omega-rich seed oil such as hemp or flax seed oil, and a squeeze of lemon juice to taste. Whizz together. Alternatively, finely chop the leaves and stir in the oil. The mixture should hold together a little like a pesto.

Superfood Salad of Quinoa with Roasted Veg

Research has shown that consuming vitamin E and the nutrient lycopene together, such as in the pumpkin seeds and tomatoes used here, enhances their positive antioxidant effects. This, combined with the zinc and protein-rich quinoa and the liver-boosting herbs, makes a superfood meal.

Serves 2

1 small sweet potato, unpeeled, cubed

1 small red onion, roughly chopped

1 red, yellow or orange pepper, deseeded and roughly chopped

1 small courgette, roughly chopped

2 garlic cloves, thinly sliced

1–2 tbsp mild olive oil

200g cherry tomatoes

150g quinoa, thoroughly rinsed

1 tsp reduced-salt vegetable bouillon powder

2 heaped tbsp pumpkin seeds

2 portions Super Greens Mix (see page 347)

1. Preheat the oven to 200°C/400°F/Gas 6. Put the chopped vegetables and garlic in a roasting tin, drizzle with oil, stir to coat, then roast for 40 minutes. Add the whole cherry tomatoes and return to the oven for a further 15–20 minutes until the tomato skins split and the sweet potatoes are soft when pierced.

2. Meanwhile, put the quinoa and bouillon powder in a pan and cover with boiling water (two parts water to one part quinoa). Bring to the boil then cover, reduce the heat and simmer for 12–15 minutes until the liquid is absorbed and the grains are fluffy. Set to one side, covered, while the vegetables finish cooking.

3. Five minutes before the vegetables are ready, put the pumpkin seeds on a baking tray and pop them in the oven on the top shelf to toast.

4. Stir the roasted vegetables and the Super Greens Mix into the quinoa, then sprinkle the toasted pumpkin seeds on top. Leave to cool or eat warm, if you prefer.

Butternut Squash and Tenderstem Broccoli Salad

Roasting brings out the flavour of butternut squash beautifully, and it tastes great tossed with salad leaves and walnuts.

🄕 if FODMAP-friendly vegetables (see page 241) are used instead of broccoli and the garlic and xylitol are omitted from the dressing.

Serves 3–4

½ butternut squash, deseeded and cut into fairly thin slices (no need to peel unless you prefer to)

2 tsp dried oregano

1–2 tbsp mild olive oil, or virgin rapeseed oil, for drizzling

200g Tenderstem broccoli

about 115g mixed leaves, such as rocket, watercress, baby spinach and lamb's lettuce

2 tbsp roughly chopped sun-dried or sun-blush tomato pieces in oil, drained

50g walnut halves, roughly chopped

For the vinaigrette dressing:

50ml extra virgin olive oil

50ml virgin pumpkin seed oil, avocado oil or rapeseed oil

15ml cider vinegar

2 tsp balsamic vinegar

1 small garlic clove, crushed

½ tsp Dijon mustard

¼ tsp xylitol

½ tsp herbes de Provence

freshly ground black pepper

1. Preheat the oven to 220°C/425°F/Gas 7. Toss the squash in the oregano and a little oil to coat, and

put on a baking tray. Roast for 25–30 minutes until tender, then set aside.

2. Steam the broccoli for 3 minutes or until just tender, then rinse in cold water to stop it cooking, and dry in a tea towel. Slice into sticks.

3. Put the leaves in a salad bowl and add the squash and broccoli. Throw in the tomato and walnut pieces.

4. Put all the vinaigrette ingredients in a blender or food processor and combine. Alternatively, put the ingredients into a screw-topped jar and shake it to emulsify them. Taste and adjust the seasoning.

5. Dress the salad with vinaigrette to taste (any leftover dressing can be stored in the refrigerator).

Gazpacho

If you would like to serve this soup in the traditional way, chilled, you can pop it into the fridge for 30 minutes–1 hour before serving, but it is also perfectly delicious eaten straight after it is made.

Serves 4
3 red, yellow or orange peppers or a mixture of colours, deseeded
1 cucumber
1 red onion
3 celery sticks
400g ripe tomatoes
2 garlic cloves, crushed
2 long, mild red chillies, deseeded (optional)
125g Peppadew sweet baby peppers, drained weight, or hot pepper or chilli sauce to taste

2 handfuls of fresh coriander
2 handfuls of flat-leaf parsley
2 ripe avocados, halved and pitted
400ml tomato juice
juice of 2 lemons
freshly ground black pepper

1. Put the peppers, cucumber, onion, celery, tomatoes, garlic, chillies (if using), Peppadew peppers, coriander and flat-leaf parsley in a food processor and process to chop finely.
2. Dice the avocado flesh and add it to the soup mixture, along with the tomato juice, lemon juice and black pepper. Stir together and adjust the seasoning to taste. If you prefer a milder flavour, don't add the Peppadew peppers or sauce, and double the amount of avocado.

Carrot and Lentil Soup

Thick and filling, this soup is perfect to keep in the fridge ready for an instant meal.

Serves 4
1 tbsp coconut oil, mild olive oil or butter
1 onion, roughly chopped
2 garlic cloves, crushed
2 large celery sticks, sliced
4 medium-large carrots, sliced
200g red split lentils, rinsed
1 litre hot vegetable stock

1. Heat the oil in a large pan over a medium heat and cook the onion for 5 minutes to soften. Add the garlic and cook gently for another 1 minute.
2. Add the celery, carrots, lentils and hot stock, then stir and bring to the boil. Reduce the heat, cover and simmer for 10 minutes to allow the carrots to soften, then blend until smooth or your preferred consistency.

Chickpea, Carrot and Coriander Soup

Grating the carrots in this delicious soup means that they soften very quickly – reducing the cooking time and any loss of nutrients.

Serves 4
400g can chickpeas, rinsed and drained
1 tbsp coconut oil, mild olive oil or butter
1 onion, finely sliced
4 carrots, coarsely grated
800ml hot vegetable stock
80g fresh coriander, fresh flat-leaf parsley or a mix of the
    two
1 tbsp extra virgin olive oil
2 tbsp lemon juice
freshly ground black pepper

1. Put the chickpeas into a food processor and blend until smooth. If necessary, add a splash of water to get a pureéd consistency.
2. Heat the coconut oil in a large pan over a medium heat and gently cook the onion for 5 minutes to soften it.

3. Stir in the carrots, then pour in the hot vegetable stock and bring to the boil. Reduce the heat, cover and simmer for 5 minutes, then add the puréed chickpeas. Return to a simmer and cook for another 5 minutes or until the carrot tastes soft and a little sweet rather than coarse and raw.
4. Meanwhile, put the herbs, olive oil and lemon juice in a blender or food processor and blitz until the herbs are finely chopped and fairly smooth.
5. Ladle the soup into bowls and put a dollop of the herb garnish in the middle before sprinkling with black pepper.

Curried Pumpkin Soup

Including spices like cumin and curry powder is a great way to boost the antioxidant content of a dish effortlessly, as they are real star performers in the antioxidant stakes. This warming, brightly coloured soup is an excellent choice if you are trying to fight off a bug or you have a sore throat.

Serves 4
1 tbsp mild olive oil, virgin rapeseed oil or coconut oil
1 large red onion, chopped
2 garlic cloves, crushed
2 tsp mild or medium curry powder
900g pumpkin or butternut squash, cut into cubes
1 large carrot, chopped
800ml hot chicken or vegetable stock
freshly ground black pepper
4 tbsp finely chopped baby spinach leaves (or blended with a little extra virgin olive or rapeseed oil)

1. Heat the oil in a large frying pan over a medium heat, add the onion, garlic and curry powder and cook for 1 minute.
2. Add the pumpkin and carrot, and cook for a further 10 minutes to pick up some colour.
3. Transfer the mixture to a large pan and add the hot stock. Bring to the boil then reduce the heat, cover and simmer for 15 minutes.
4. Blend until smooth, then season with pepper to taste. Ladle the soup into bowls, then place a spoonful of the chopped spinach in the middle of each bowl.

Broccoli Soup

This is much better tasting than its simple ingredients would suggest, so do give it a try. It is a quick and easy way to increase your intake of greens.

Serves 2
1 tbsp mild olive oil, virgin rapeseed oil or coconut oil
2 garlic cloves, crushed
500ml hot vegetable stock
400g broccoli, cut into florets
100ml milk or non-dairy milk such as coconut milk or oat, rice or soya milk
freshly ground black pepper

1. Heat the oil in a large pan over a medium heat, add the garlic and gently cook for 1 minute, taking care not to let it burn.
2. Add the hot stock and the broccoli, and bring to the boil.

3. Reduce the heat, cover and simmer for 10 minutes or until the broccoli is tender.
4. Add the milk and plenty of black pepper, then blend until smooth. Adjust the seasoning if necessary.

Coconut Milk and Mushroom Broth

This Asian-inspired broth is wonderfully soothing if you are feeling under the weather, and the coconut milk lends a creamy smoothness. This recipe serves two because it is best made fresh, but by all means increase the quantities to feed more.

Serves 2
700ml hot chicken or vegetable stock
200ml coconut milk
½ tbsp tamari or soy sauce
½ tbsp Thai fish sauce
1–2 tsp Thai tom yum paste, to taste
1 tsp xylitol or coconut palm sugar
6 very thin slices peeled galangal or ginger
15g mixed dried wild or shiitake mushrooms, soaked for 20 minutes and drained, sliced

1. Pour the hot stock into a pan over high heat and bring to the boil. Add the coconut milk and boil the mixture for 5 minutes.
2. Lower the heat to a gentle simmer, and then add the tamari, fish sauce, tom yum paste, xylitol, galangal and the mushrooms. Leave the soup to simmer, uncovered, for 20 minutes or until the mushrooms have softened. Taste to check the seasoning before serving.

Dinners

Vegetarian

Baked Sweet Potatoes with Borlotti Stew

Sweet potatoes are incredibly rich in the antioxidant vitamins beta-carotene and vitamin E, both of which are required to keep the immune system functioning and to keep skin, both inside and out, in good condition. They are deliciously smooth and sweet when baked, and make a very filling, warming meal when topped with this rich, thick ragout-style bean stew.

Serves 2
2 large sweet potatoes
a little medium (not extra virgin) olive oil
For the stew:
1 tbsp coconut oil or olive oil
2 garlic cloves, crushed
1 large red onion, diced
100g mushrooms, sliced
2 tbsp tomato purée
400g can plum tomatoes
400g can borlotti beans, rinsed and drained
½ tsp reduced-salt vegetable bouillon powder
½ tsp herbes de Provence, or to taste
freshly ground black pepper

1. Preheat the oven to 200°C/400°F/Gas 6. Prick the potatoes all over. Rub with a little oil and put on a baking tray. Bake for 1 hour or until soft all the way through when pierced with a knife.

2. Meanwhile, prepare the stew. Heat the oil in a pan over a medium heat and cook the garlic and onion gently for 2 minutes, then add the mushrooms and cook for 5 minutes or until fairly soft.

3. Add the remaining ingredients and simmer for 5–10 minutes to allow the vegetables to soften and the sauce to thicken. Check the seasoning and adjust if necessary.

4. Open up the baked potatoes and spoon the stew inside.

Fennel and Mixed Rice Pilaff

Fennel is an excellent liver booster and the wild rice (which is actually a grass) provides more protein and minerals than standard rice. The recipe is delicious cold, so you can eat this for supper and then take some to work the next day for lunch. Serve with a mixed leaf salad.

Serves 2
1 tsp reduced-salt vegetable bouillon powder
90g mixed rice (wild rice, brown basmati rice and red Camargue rice)
1 tbsp coconut oil or mild olive oil
1 small or ½ large red onion, peeled and cut into thin wedges
½ fennel bulb, thinly sliced lengthways
115g chestnut mushrooms, quartered
400g can green lentils, rinsed and drained
1 tbsp lemon juice
2 tbsp finely chopped fresh flat-leaf parsley
freshly ground black pepper

1. Bring a large pan of water to the boil and add the bouillon powder. Cook the rice according to the pack instructions. As the grains are unrefined they should be tender when cooked but still retain some bite. Drain the rice.
2. While the rice is cooking, heat the oil in a large frying pan over a medium heat and cook the onion, fennel and mushrooms over a medium-high heat for 5–10 minutes until softened. Reduce the heat while you prepare the rice.
3. Add the rice to the pan of vegetables along with the lentils, and stir over a medium-low heat. Add the lemon juice, parsley and lots of black pepper. Taste to check the seasoning before serving.

Rice with Super Greens Pesto

A cross between a pesto and a tapenade, the combination of olives and herbs in the sauce for this dish adds flavour and texture as well as topping up your nutrient levels. Serve with a large mixed salad.

Serves 2
150g brown basmati rice, rinsed
2 portions of Super Greens Mix (see page 347)
2 tbsp pumpkin seeds, lightly toasted for 2 minutes in a dry frying pan until they start to swell and pop
6 tbsp pitted Kalamata olives
2 tbsp extra virgin olive oil (from the jar if the olives are stored in oil)
2 large garlic cloves, crushed
4 handfuls of fresh basil leaves
2 handfuls of rocket

2 handfuls of baby spinach or fresh flat-leaf parsley leaves
freshly ground black pepper
juice of 1 lemon, or to taste

1. Cook the rice according to the instructions on the packet (usually about 20 minutes).
2. Meanwhile, to prepare the Super Greens pesto, whizz all the remaining ingredients together in a mini blender or food processor. Taste to check the flavour – you can add more of any of the ingredients to tweak the flavour, if you like. Toss the pesto through the rice. Serve warm.

Mushroom and Pine Nut Stuffed Peppers

Peppers are very high in antioxidants and vitamin C. They are delicious served here stuffed with a rich rice mixture of pine nuts, basil and mushrooms. To make this even healthier, choose shiitake mushrooms for their lentinan content, as this polysaccharide is a powerful immune booster long used in traditional Chinese medicine.

Serves 2
2 large red peppers
1 tbsp coconut oil or mild olive oil
1 medium onion, finely chopped
2 garlic cloves, crushed
150g mushrooms, sliced
1 tsp reduced-salt vegetable bouillon powder
115g brown basmati rice, cooked, 50g raw weight
1 tbsp pine nuts
a fresh basil, chopped

1. Preheat the oven to 200°C/400°F/Gas 6. Cut the tops off the peppers (reserving them to make lids) and remove the seeds and pith.
2. Heat the oil in a pan over a medium heat and gently fry the onion and garlic for 2 minutes. Add the mushrooms and bouillon powder and cook for a further 2–3 minutes.
3. Transfer to a large bowl and add the cooked rice, nuts and basil.
4. Stuff the peppers with the mixture and put the tops back on.
5. Put on a baking tray and bake for 35 minutes.

Chickpea and Cauliflower Curry

The turmeric in this curry gives it anti-inflammatory properties to offer relief from allergy symptoms. When you buy the coconut milk, don't get a reduced-fat version, as many of coconut's renowned health properties are due to its medium-chain triglycerides, which are easier to burn for energy than to store as fat.

Serves 4
2 tbsp coconut oil or mild or medium (not extra virgin) olive oil
3 tbsp medium curry paste
2 large onions, sliced
½ cauliflower, broken into small florets
400g can chickpeas, rinsed and drained
400ml can coconut milk
210ml hot vegetable stock
1 tbsp tamari or soy sauce
250g fine green beans
a handful of fresh coriander, leaves torn or roughly chopped

1. Put the oil and the curry paste in a large frying pan or wok over a medium heat and add the onions, then cook for 5 minutes to soften them. Add the cauliflower and chickpeas to the pan, and stir to coat them in the other ingredients.
2. Pour in the coconut milk, stock and tamari, and stir. Bring to the boil, then cover and simmer over a gentle heat for 30 minutes or until the cauliflower is fairly soft.
3. Stir in the green beans and cook for another 5 minutes or until they are tender. Scatter with the coriander leaves before serving.

Lentil Dhal

This Indian staple is traditionally served as a milder accompaniment to curries, but if you add plenty of spices, garlic and ginger, it is very good served on its own with rice and perhaps some finely diced red onion, tomato and cucumber.

Serves 4
1 tbsp virgin rapeseed oil or coconut oil
1 tsp ground turmeric
1 tsp ground cumin
2 tsp garam masala
1 garlic clove, crushed
1 red onion, diced
2cm fresh root ginger, peeled and grated
1 medium carrot, diced or thinly sliced
165g red lentils, rinsed and drained
750ml vegetable stock
1 medium sweet potato, cut into small cubes
2 handfuls baby spinach, shredded

juice of ½ lemon
freshly ground black pepper

1. Heat the oil in a large frying pan over a medium heat, add the spices, garlic, onion and ginger and fry for 1 minute. Add the carrot and lentils, stir and pour in the stock.
2. Bring to the boil, then fast boil for 10 minutes before reducing the heat to a simmer. Add the sweet potato, stir, and cook for 15 minutes or until the lentils and sweet potato are soft.
3. Stir in the spinach and let it wilt, then add the lemon juice and season with pepper to taste before serving.

Wild Rice and Puy Lentils with Lemon and Asparagus

Rich in protein and minerals, wild rice is a grass and not in fact a rice. Accompany this dish with a red onion, tomato, avocado and basil salad.

Serves 6
250g wild rice
150g dried Puy lentils
1 tsp reduced-salt vegetable bouillon powder
2 courgettes, thinly sliced lengthways
8 spring onions, trimmed
200g fine asparagus spears
juice of 2 lemons, plus the zest and juice of 2 organic or
    unwaxed lemons
4 tbsp mild or medium (not extra virgin) olive oil
4 tbsp extra virgin olive oil
freshly ground black pepper

1. Put the rice and lentils in a large pan and pour boiling water over them. Cover and soak for 4 hours to soften and reduce the cooking time. Drain off the soaked rice and lentils, return to the pan with the vegetable bouillon and re-cover with 600ml boiling water. Bring to the boil, then cover and simmer for 20 minutes or until cooked and the water has been absorbed.

2. Meanwhile, put the courgettes in a large bowl with the spring onions and asparagus, and pour the juice of 2 lemons and the mild olive oil over them, stirring to coat. Leave to marinate for at least 10 minutes.

3. Preheat a griddle pan over a medium-high heat until smoking, then griddle the courgette slices very quickly in batches, turning them over to colour on both sides. Add each cooked batch to the pan of cooked rice and lentils. Then griddle the spring onions for 4–5 minutes, rolling occasionally to colour evenly, then put with the rice and lentils. Next, put the asparagus on the griddle pan – you will probably have to do this in batches – and cook for 5 minutes, rolling occasionally to cook evenly. Pour a few tablespoons of the leftover marinade into the griddle pan to par-steam the asparagus for a further 1–2 minutes until soft. Transfer the asparagus to the rice and lentils.

4. Fold the griddled vegetables into the rice and lentils, along with the zest and juice of the remaining 2 lemons, the extra virgin olive oil, black pepper to taste. Serve warm or at room temperature.

Fish

Trout en Papillote with Roasted Vegetables

Cooking fish en papillote (in a parcel of baking paper) pre-
serves all of its juices, flavour and essential fats.

F if the garlic is omitted.

Serves 2

2 medium or 1 large sweet potato, sliced into fairly thin
    wedges
2 courgettes, sliced into similar-sized wedges
a drizzle of mild olive oil
2 medium-sized rainbow trout (preferably organic), fully
    prepared
2 garlic cloves, crushed
juice of 1 lemon
2 tsp finely chopped fresh flat-leaf parsley leaves
2 portions of Super Greens Mix (see page 347)

1. Preheat the oven to 180°C/350°F/Gas 4. Put the
    sweet potatoes and courgettes in a roasting tin,
    drizzle with the oil and roast for 1 hour, turning
    the vegetables over halfway through, until the
    sweet potatoes are soft when pierced with a knife.
2. Meanwhile, cut a piece of baking paper large
    enough to cover both fish lying diagonally across
    the middle of the paper when folded in half on the
    diagonal.
3. Season the inside of each fish with the garlic,
    lemon juice and parsley, and put the fish diagonally
    across the baking parchment then fold in half on
    the diagonal.

4. Starting from one end, gradually fold up the edges to seal the paper into a parcel, overlapping each fold slightly over the last fold to stop it unravelling.
5. Put the parcel on a baking tray and bake for 25 minutes. Unwrap carefully to avoid being scalded by the steam, and put the fish on plates with the cooked vegetables and a portion of Super Greens Mix each. Serve immediately.

Salmon with Puy Lentils

Steaming the salmon helps to preserve as much of the valuable omega-3 fats as possible, because it is a much gentler cooking technique than the direct, fierce heat from a frying pan or grill. This dish is also delicious cold.

Serves 2
115g Puy lentils, rinsed and drained
2 tsp reduced-salt vegetable bouillon powder
2 leeks, finely sliced
2 salmon fillets (preferably organic)
2 tbsp tomato purée
a squeeze of fresh lemon juice
2 portions of Super Greens Mix (see page 347)
freshly ground black pepper

1. Put the lentils in a pan and cover with double the amount of water by volume. Add the bouillon powder. Bring to the boil then cover and simmer for 15 minutes. Add the leeks and continue cooking for 10–15 minutes or until the lentils are al dente (firm to the bite). The lentils will absorb most of the liquid during cooking.

2. Put the salmon in a steamer pan over a high
   heat and steam for 15 minutes or until cooked –
   the flesh should flake easily when pressed.
   (Alternatively, if you don't have a steamer, put the
   fish in a frying pan over a medium heat, cover with
   water and simmer gently until the flesh flakes when
   pressed.)
3. Stir the tomato purée into the lentil mixture along
   with a splash of water and the lemon juice to
   loosen the consistency and produce a thick stew.
4. Either serve the salmon on a bed of stew and
   scatter the Super Greens Mix over the top, or fold
   the greens mixture into the stew before topping
   with the fish. Sprinkle with freshly ground black
   pepper.

Kedgeree

To keep this dish low in GLs this kedgeree is lower on rice
than a regular kedgeree, but it's full of flavour, filling and
contains plenty of digestion-friendly ingredients.

Serves 4
180g brown basmati rice
275g mackerel fillets
2 organic or free-range eggs
200g Tenderstem broccoli
115g frozen petits pois
2 tbsp mild, medium (not extra virgin) olive oil
1 garlic clove, crushed
2 small red onions, finely chopped
1 tbsp mild curry powder
1 tsp ground turmeric

4 tbsp finely chopped flat-leaf parsley
freshly ground black pepper
lemons wedges, to serve

1. Cook the rice according to the pack instructions, then drain and set aside until ready to use.
2. Meanwhile, fill a large frying pan with water and bring to a gentle boil. Put the mackerel in the pan, making sure it is covered by the liquid, and gently poach for 4–6 minutes or until the flesh flakes easily when pressed. Carefully remove the fish from the pan and leave to cool. Then remove the skin and flake into pieces, picking out any bones.
3. Hard-boil the eggs in a pan of boiling water for 6 minutes, then cool rapidly under the tap for 1 minute. Set aside to cool fully before peeling and slicing into quarters.
4. Steam the Tenderstem broccoli and petits pois for 3 minutes, then slice the Tenderstem into lengths of about 2.5cm.
5. Add the oil to a large pan over a medium heat and cook the garlic and onions for 1 minute, then add the spices. Cook gently for 3 minutes, or until the onions are soft and fragrant, taking care not to let the spices burn.
6. Stir the cooked rice into the onion and spice mixture until evenly coated. Gently fold in the fish, Tenderstem, peas and hard-boiled eggs.
7. Season with plenty of pepper. Add the parsley and stir carefully. Taste to check the seasoning and serve with a lemon wedge on each plate.

Tandoori Fish

The herbs and spices used to marinate the fish in this recipe help to tenderise the flesh and add plenty of flavour. They are also long-acknowledged digestion and immune system boosters.

Serves 4

2 tsp garam masala
1 tsp ground cumin
1 tsp ground coriander
1 tsp ground turmeric
1cm fresh root ginger, peeled and grated
1 garlic clove, crushed
2 tbsp finely chopped fresh coriander
juice of half a lemon
6 tbsp natural yoghurt
4 × 150g line-caught cod loin fillets, boned and skinned
freshly ground black pepper

1. Make the marinade by mixing all the ingredients, except the fish and pepper, in a large bowl.
2. Coat the fish completely in the marinade. Cover and put in the fridge for at least 30 minutes or up to 60 minutes – be careful not to leave the fish in the marinade for too long, though, as the lemon juice might turn it mushy.
3. Preheat the grill to medium-high, then grill the fish for 15 minutes, turning it halfway through, or until the flesh flakes easily when pressed. Sprinkle with black pepper and serve immediately, taking care not to break the fillets when you transfer the fish to the plates.

Sea Bass with Braised Fennel and Roast New Potatoes

Fish and fennel are a flavour marriage made in heaven. Fennel is considered to be very beneficial to the liver, aiding detoxification.

Serves 4
4 sea bass fillets, 125g each
1 tbsp mild olive oil
freshly ground black pepper
1 lemon, sliced into wedges, to serve
For the roast potatoes:
700g baby new potatoes
a drizzle of mild olive oil
For the braised fennel:
1 tbsp mild olive oil
2 fennel bulbs, tough outer leaves and stalks removed, sliced
50ml vegetable stock

1. Preheat the oven to 180°C/350°F/Gas 4. To make the roast potatoes, cut any large potatoes so that they are all a similar size. Put the potatoes in a roasting tin, drizzle with the oil and shake the tin to coat the potatoes evenly. Cook for 1 hour, turning them halfway through the cooking time.
2. Meanwhile, make the braised fennel. Heat the oil in a pan over a medium heat, add the fennel slices and cook for 6–8 minutes until they start to soften. Add the stock and braise for 15 minutes or until very soft.
3. When the potatoes are ready, heat the oil in a large frying pan over a medium-high heat and fry the fish for 4–6 minutes, turning halfway through when the bottom is starting to look white and

cooked, to make the skin crisp. Don't get distracted at this stage, as over-cooking the fish will ruin the delicate texture and flavour.

4. Serve immediately, with the potatoes and fennel. Pour over a little of the fennel braising liquor, if there is any left over, and add lots of black pepper. Serve with lemon wedges to squeeze over.

Thai Fishcakes

These light, highly flavoured, Oriental-style fishcakes are packed with nutritious superfoods.

Serves 4
4 garlic cloves, crushed
2 large mild, red chillies, deseeded (optional)
5cm fresh root ginger, peeled and grated
4 spring onions
grated zest of 2 limes
4 tbsp chopped fresh coriander
4 tbsp tamari, soy sauce or fish sauce
2 tbsp toasted sesame oil
500g salmon, haddock, cod or hake fillet, skinned and
     boned, cut into 4 pieces
4 tbsp cornflour
1 tbsp coconut oil or mild olive oil
For the dipping sauce:
2 tbsp toasted sesame oil
2 tbsp tamari or soy sauce
juice of 2 limes
8 spring onions, finely chopped
4 tbsp finely chopped fresh coriander
2 tbsp sesame seeds, lightly toasted in a dry frying pan

1. Put the garlic, chillies (if using), ginger, spring onions, lime zest and coriander into a food processor with the tamari and sesame oil, and blend to combine. Add the fish and blend until the mixture is finely chopped but not entirely smooth.
2. Shape the mixture into 12 patties, squash them down into flat circles and dust them lightly with cornflour. Put them in the fridge to firm up.
3. To make the dipping sauce, put the oil in a bowl and add the tamari, lime juice, spring onions and coriander. Mix together until smooth, then stir in the sesame seeds.
4. Heat the coconut oil in a large frying pan or wok over a medium-high heat and fry the fishcakes for 3–4 minutes on each side until golden. You will need to do this in batches. Drain on kitchen paper and serve with the dipping sauce.

Steamed Trout with Ginger

The addition of chilli, ginger, garlic and lime makes a simple steamed fish dish much more interesting, as well as contributing antioxidants and myriad other health benefits. Try serving this dish with brown basmati rice or soba (buckwheat) noodles tossed with toasted sesame seeds.

❶ if spring onions and garlic are omitted.

Serves 2
2 trout fillets, each weighing about 140g
115g baby pak choi, each quartered lengthways
3 spring onions, finely sliced on the diagonal
1 small garlic clove, crushed

1cm fresh root ginger, grated
1 tsp very finely chopped, deseeded red chilli (optional)
grated zest and juice of 1 lime
2 tbsp tamari or soy sauce
1 tbsp toasted sesame oil

1. Cut a large rectangle of baking paper and put it into a steamer pan, then put the fish fillets next to each other in the middle of the paper.
2. Put the pak choi around the edge of the fish and scatter the spring onions over the top.
3. Put the garlic in a bowl and add the ginger, chilli (if using), lime zest and juice, tamari and sesame oil. Mix well together, then pour over the fish and vegetables.
4. Bring the edges of the paper together in the middle and fold over to loosely seal. Steam the parcel for 15 minutes.
5. Open the parcel carefully, check that the fish is cooked by pressing it to see if it flakes easily, then serve.

Steamed Salmon with Soy and Garlic Spring Greens

Steaming is perhaps the healthiest method of all for cooking oily fish, as it is so gentle on the delicate essential fats.
🅕 if spring onions and garlic are omitted.

Serves 2
2 salmon fillets, about 110g each
2 tsp tamari or soy sauce
2 tbsp coconut oil, or virgin rapeseed oil
6 spring onions, very finely sliced lengthways

For the spring greens:

2 tbsp virgin rapeseed oil or coconut oil

2 garlic cloves, lightly crushed using the back of the knife
and kept whole

2 small heads of spring greens, thinly sliced

2 tsp tamari or soy sauce, or to taste

1. Put the salmon in a steamer pan over a high
heat and steam for 10–14 minutes until cooked –
the flesh should flake easily when pressed.
(Alternatively, if you don't have a steamer, put the
fish in a frying pan, cover with water and simmer
gently until the flesh flakes when pressed.)

2. Meanwhile, to make the spring greens, put the oil
in a hot wok or frying pan over a medium heat.
Add the garlic and stir-fry for 15 seconds, then
add the greens and stir-fry for 2 minutes to soften
slightly. Add the tamari, then set to one side as you
quickly serve the fish.

3. Put the salmon fillets onto two plates and drizzle
with a teaspoon of tamari.

4. Heat the oil in a frying pan over a medium-high
heat until very hot, then throw in the spring onions
and cook for 1 minute just to wilt. Spoon the
spring onions over each piece of salmon.

Pan-fried Pollack and Sweet Potato Chips

This is a healthier take on the great British takeaway. Sweet
potato appears to help your body regulate blood sugar levels,
making it a much better choice for your chips than ordinary
white potatoes. Serve with a green leaf salad or some wilted
spinach.

Serves 2

2 pollack fillets, about 150g each, preferably with skin on

1 tbsp mild olive oil or virgin rapeseed oil

freshly ground black pepper

2 lemon wedges, to serve

For the chips:

1 medium-large sweet potato, cut into chips

1 tbsp mild or medium olive oil or virgin rapeseed oil

1. Preheat the oven to 180°C/350°F/Gas 4. To make the chips, put the sweet potato chips in a large bowl and toss with the oil. Spread out in a shallow roasting tin and roast for 30–40 minutes until crisp.

2. Heat the oil in a frying pan over a medium-high heat, then put the fish in the pan, skin-side down. Cook the fish for 2 minutes or until the fillets are opaque almost all the way through. Turn the fish over and carry on cooking until the fish has coloured all the way through (this will only take another 1 minute or so).

3. Put the fish on plates with the sweet potato chips and season with black pepper. Serve with a lemon wedge.

Chicken

Chicken Satay Skewers

This Eastern-style satay sauce is packed with healthy ingredients from the ginger, garlic and onion to the chilli, lemon and coriander. Serve with quinoa or brown basmati rice.

Serves 4

500g skinless, boneless chicken thigh fillets, cut into bite-
sized pieces

2 tbsp medium or mild (not extra virgin) olive oil

1 tbsp tamari or soy sauce

For the satay sauce:

4 tbsp peanuts or cashew nuts, lightly toasted in a dry frying
pan and finely chopped

4 tbsp sugar-free crunchy peanut butter

2 tbsp groundnut oil or untoasted sesame oil

2 tbsp water

2 garlic cloves, crushed

6cm fresh root ginger, peeled and grated

1 tbsp finely chopped mild red chilli (optional)

4 tbsp finely chopped fresh coriander

4 spring onions, very finely sliced

1–2 tsp tamari or soy sauce, to taste

2–3 tbsp toasted sesame oil, to taste

juice of 1 lemon or 2 limes

1. To make the satay sauce, put all the ingredients,
   except the toasted sesame oil and lemon, in a
   bowl and mix well. (Alternatively, if you want to
   save time on the chopping and grating, whizz the
   ingredients together in a blender or food processor.)
   Then add the reserved oil and juice little by little,
   testing for consistency and taste. Spoon the sauce
   into a small bowl.
2. Preheat the grill to high. Put the chicken in a bowl,
   drizzle with the oil and tamari, and mix to coat.
   Thread the chicken on to skewers.
3. Grill the chicken for 10 minutes, turning
   occasionally so that it cooks evenly, or until the

meat is cooked through and the juices run clear. Divide the skewers between four plates and invite guests to help themselves to the sauce.

Moroccan-Style Chicken

This recipe is particularly good served with Kamut pasta which has proven IBS friendly in a clinical trial, unlike modern wheat.

Serves 4
1 tbsp coconut oil or mild or medium (not extra virgin) olive oil
2 red onions, sliced
4 skinless organic or free-range chicken breasts, cubed
700g butternut squash, unpeeled, deseeded, cubed
1 tsp ground cinnamon
1 tsp ground ginger
1 tsp ground turmeric
1 litre chicken stock
chopped fresh coriander and mint, for sprinkling
freshly ground black pepper

1. Heat the oil in a large pan over a medium heat and cook the onions for 3–4 minutes. Add the chicken, squash and spices, and stir for 2 minutes.
2. Pour in the stock, bring to the boil, then cover and simmer for 30 minutes. Uncover and simmer for a further 10 minutes to allow the meat to cook fully (the juices should run clear) and the sauce to thicken. Sprinkle with coriander, mint and black pepper before serving.

Chicken and Puy Lentil One-pot Stew

Puy lentils are the only type of lentil to hold their shape once cooked, avoiding the mushy consistency that puts many people off pulses. This hearty stew is a balanced meal on its own, but you could also serve it with some steamed savoy cabbage or spring greens, or some mashed sweet potato.

Serves 4

2 tbsp coconut oil, or medium or mild (not extra virgin) olive
    oil or virgin rapeseed oil
16 shallots, peeled and left whole, or 4 large red onions, cut
    into wedges
4 garlic cloves, crushed
250g button mushrooms
4 tsp ground coriander
4 tsp ground cumin
2.5cm piece of fresh root ginger, grated
8 tbsp tomato purée
2 carrots, thinly sliced
2 celery sticks, sliced
1 litre hot chicken stock
200g dried Puy lentils
4 large chicken thighs, or 8 smaller thigh fillets, skinned
freshly ground black pepper

1. Heat the oil in a large pan over a medium heat and add the onions, garlic and mushrooms. Cook gently for 5 minutes, then stir in the ground coriander, cumin and ginger and cook for 2 minutes.
2. Stir in the tomato purée and add the carrots, celery, hot stock, lentils and the chicken to the pan. Stir to

ensure that the chicken is submerged in the liquid, then cover.

3. Simmer for 35 minutes, then uncover and simmer for a further 15 minutes or until the sauce is thickened and the chicken cooked through (the juices must run clear).

4. Season with pepper to taste.

Thai Chicken and Cashew Stir-fry

Serve with brown basmati rice or soba (buckwheat) noodles, and perhaps some stir-fried veg. You can get holy basil leaves from Chinese supermarkets (don't substitute ordinary basil, as the flavour is very different).

Serves 2

2 garlic cloves

2 small red chillies, deseeded (optional, but this is a fundamental part of the recipe)

1 tbsp mild-flavoured oil such as rapeseed oil or coconut oil

2 skinless chicken breasts, cut into thin strips

8 spring onions, trimmed and cut into 2.5cm strips on the diagonal

115g roasted, unsalted cashew nuts

1 tsp xylitol or coconut palm sugar

2 tsp soy sauce or tamari

1½ tbsp fish sauce

3 tbsp chicken stock

15 holy basil leaves, shredded

1 tbsp Thai chilli paste

1. Crush the garlic and chillies (if using) to a paste using a mortar and pestle. Heat the wok over a

medium heat, then add the oil and swirl to coat the wok.

2. Add the garlic and chilli paste and the chicken, and cook for 2–3 minutes until the chicken is cooked through.

3. Add the spring onions and cook for 30 seconds, then add the cashew nuts and cook for another 30 seconds.

4. Add the xylitol, soy sauce and fish sauce. Stir well, then add the stock.

5. Add the basil leaves and chilli paste, then stir before serving.

CHAPTER 34

Gut-Friendly Snacks

Provided you don't have candida, eating a small amount of a low-GL fruit, such as berries, an apple or pear, with some live natural yoghurt or soya yoghurt and a handful of unroasted, unsalted nuts or seeds makes a very good snack. Another favourite is oatcakes with a suitable spread such as hummus, taramasalata, a little smoked salmon, or a nut butter. Try making your own hummus and guacamole from the recipes below, to have with oatcakes or crudités, such as a raw carrot.

NOTE ❶ = FODMAP friendly

Provided you don't have candida, a small amount of fruit that is low GL (see page 53), such as berries, apples or pears, and some live natural yoghurt and unsalted nuts, is a very good snack. Another good choice is oatcakes with a spread such as hummus, guacamole or nut butter, or a little smoked salmon. Try making your own spreads from the recipes in this section.

Guacamole

This is great with crudités, but don't just stick to the usual carrot, celery and cucumber crudités; try sugar snap peas, baby corn, white cabbage, radishes, spring onions, celeriac, peppers, cherry tomatoes and fennel.

Serves 2
1 ripe avocado, halved and pitted
juice of ¼ lemon
½ garlic clove, crushed
¼ small red onion, finely diced
3 cherry tomatoes, finely diced
1 tbsp chopped fresh coriander and/or fresh flat-leaf parsley (optional)
1 tbsp extra virgin olive oil, or omega-rich seed oil like flax seed (linseed), hemp or pumpkin seed oil (optional)
freshly ground black pepper

Scrape the flesh out of the avocado shell into a bowl and add the remaining ingredients. Quickly mash together, then season with pepper to taste. (Keep any leftovers covered in the fridge for up to two days.)

Corn on the Cob

This is a very filling snack, and the bright yellow corn kernels are packed with beta-carotene, an essential antioxidant. Most people slather corn on the cob in butter, but corn has so much natural sweetness and juiciness that you don't need anything on it other than perhaps a splash of lemon juice.

F if well cooked.

Serves 1
1 corn on the cob
lemon juice to drizzle (optional)

1. Cut off the stalk end of the cob and peel away the outer husk and silk. Trim off the pointed end. Put a couple of sheets of kitchen paper on a large plate.
2. Bring a pan of water to the boil then put the cob in the pan and boil for 5–15 minutes until a kernel of corn comes away easily.
3. Remove from the pan and put the cob on the kitchen paper to absorb any excess moisture. You can drizzle with lemon juice if you like. Eat with your fingers or use corn skewers.

Roasted Pumpkin Seeds

Seeds make a healthy topping for salads or rice dishes and are particularly tasty when roasted.

50g pumpkin seeds

Heat a dry frying pan over a medium heat and add the pumpkin seeds. Cook for 2 minutes, tossing the seeds in the pan occasionally, until they start to pop and go golden. Remove from the pan immediately and leave to cool. Store in an airtight container.

Baked Falafel

This traditional Middle Eastern dish is spicy and full of flavour as well as being packed with digestion-friendly ingredients.

Serves 4

2 × 400g cans chickpeas, rinsed and drained, or 275g dried
   chickpeas, soaked overnight and cooked, then drained
4 garlic cloves, crushed
4 tsp tahini
10 spring onions, roughly sliced
50g sesame seeds
4 tsp ground cumin
2 tsp ground coriander
2 tbsp fresh flat-leaf parsley, finely chopped
2 organic or free-range eggs, beaten
60g sesame seeds, for coating
freshly ground black pepper

1. Preheat the oven to 200°C/400°F/Gas 6. Line a
   baking tray with non-stick baking paper. Put the
   chickpeas, garlic, tahini, spring onions, sesame
   seeds, spices and parsley in a food processor and
   blend until fairly smooth and combined. Season
   with pepper to taste. Mix in the egg and shape into
   16 golf ball-sized balls.
2. Put the sesame seeds on a plate and roll the balls
   in them. This is a bit fiddly, so you might prefer
   to scatter the seeds over each side of the falafel. It
   might be necessary to then reshape the falafel in
   your hand.
3. Put the balls on the prepared baking tray and cook
   in the oven for 20–25 minutes until just golden on
   the top and firm to the touch.

Hummus

A classic Middle Eastern staple, hummus is rich in fibre and antioxidants from the garlic, tahini and lemon juice. This version cuts down on the oil and salt content compared to standard versions without compromising on flavour.

Serves 4
400g can chickpeas in water, rinsed and drained
juice of ½ lemon
1 large garlic clove, crushed
1 tbsp tahini
75ml extra virgin olive oil, or a little extra if needed
freshly ground black pepper

Blend all the ingredients together until smooth and creamy. If you want a smoother consistency, add an extra drizzle of olive oil or a splash of water. Taste and adjust the seasoning.

Blueberry Yoghurt Sundae

If you have digestive problems, try sheep's or goat's milk yoghurt, as they tend to be better tolerated than cow's milk.

Serves 1
3 heaped tbsp blueberries
3 heaped tbsp live natural yoghurt or sheep's or goat's
4 tsp ground chia seeds, or other seeds or flaked almonds
2 squirts of Cherry Active juice, or blueberry juice

Put the blueberries into a wide glass or a dessert bowl. Spoon the yoghurt over the berries, then scatter the seeds or almonds over the top. Finish by drizzling the juice over the top.

Recommended Reading

Axe, Josh, *Eat Dirt*, Bluebird, 2016

Baker, Sidney MacDonald, *Detoxification and Healing*, Keats Publishing, 1997

Bland, Jeffrey, *The 20-Day Rejuvenation Diet Programme*, Keats Publishing, 1997

Brown, Benjamin, *The Digestive Health Solution*, Exisle Publishing, 2015

Cannon, Geoffrey, *Superbug: Nature's Revenge – Why Antibiotics Can Breed Disease*, Virgin, 1999

Crook, Dr William, *The Yeast Connection*, Vintage Books, 1986

Galland, Dr Leo, *Power Healing*, Random House, 1998

Holford, Patrick, *10 Secrets of 100% Healthy People*, Piatkus, 2009

Holford, Patrick, *100% Health Cookbook*, Piatkus, 2012

Holford, Patrick and Fiona McDonald Joyce, *Delicious, Healthy, Sugar-Free*, Piatkus, 2017

Holford, Patrick and Fiona McDonald Joyce, *The 9-Day Liver Detox*, Piatkus, 2007

Holford, Patrick, *The Feel Good Factor*, Piatkus, 2010

Holford, Patrick, *The Chemistry of Connection*, Hay House, 2016

Holford, Patrick, *The Optimum Nutrition Bible*, Piatkus, 1997

Holford, Patrick and Judy Ridgway, *The Optimum Nutrition Cookbook*, Piatkus, 1999

Holford, Patrick and Susannah Lawson, *The Stress Cure*, Piatkus, 2015

Lipski, Elizabeth, *Digestive Wellness*, McGraw-Hill Education, 2011

White, Erica, *The Beat Candida Cookbook*, Thorsons, revised edition, 2011

Resources

Colonic therapists To find a registered colonic hydrotherapist, visit www.colonic-association.org/.

Digestion-friendly supplements

BioCare produce a wide range of supplements specialising in probiotics, including glutamine powder. Tel: 0121 433 3727; website: www.BioCare.co.uk.

Higher Nature produce a wide range of products, including betaine hydrochloride. Tel: 0800 458 4747; website www.highernature.co.uk.

Viridian produce a range of digestive enzymes and probiotics, including *Saccharomyces boulardii*, as well as betaine hydrochloride. Available from health food shops and www.viridian-nutrition.com.

Patrick Holford supplements, including Digestpro (a combination of digestive enzymes, probiotics and glutamine), are available from www.HOLFORDirect.com and good health-food shops.

100% Health Check You can have your own personal health and nutrition assessment online using Patrick Holford's 100% Health Check. This gives you a personalised assessment of your current health, and what you most need to change. You will also be given a personalised supplement programme. With regard to candida, ideally, your nutritional status should be monitored and the supplement programme reassessed at three-monthly intervals. The 100% Health Check can work this out for you. Visit www. patrickholford.com.

Heartmath Visit www.heartmath.co.uk for details of events, training, HeartMath coaches and products. If you are looking for research and related information, go to www.heartmath.org or www.heartmath.co.uk. For the Quick Coherence Technique go to www.patrickholford.com/heartmath. You can also learn the Quick Coherence Technique by watching a film at www.patrickholford. com/cennection/comingfromtheheart.

Homocysteine For advice on how to lower your homocysteine level, go to www.patrickholford.com/advice/how-to-lower-your-homocysteine-level.

Kamut® khorasan This ancient form of wheat is becoming more widely available in many organic and health-food shops and bakeries in Europe. In the UK, Doves Farm Foods, sells organic Kamut khorasan wholemeal flour online from www.dovesfarm.com. Kamut pasta and bulgar are available from www.HOLFORDirect. com. Visit www.Kamut.com, and select your country, to see a full list of what is available. In the UK, M&S, for example, has a Kamut spaghetti and Tesco has introduced a quick-cook grain that you cook for 10 minutes and eat like rice. A growing number of bakeries are making Kamut bread, and Infinity Foods sell a Kamut muesli.

Kefir suppliers For starting your colony of kefir and for everything need to own or know about kefir, visit www.happykombucha.co.uk.

Nutritional therapists The British Association for Applied Nutrition & Therapy (BANT) has a list of nutritional therapists. Tel: 0870 606 1284 or visit www.bant.org.uk. In Ireland see the Nutritional Therapist of Ireland at www.ntoi.ie and in South Africa see the South African Association of Nutritional Therapists at www.saant.org.za.

Psychocalisthenics exercises Psychocalisthenics is an excellent exercise system that takes less than 20 minutes a day, and develops strength, suppleness and stamina, as well as generating vital energy. For further information, see www.pcals.com. For training in the UK, visit www.integralview.org and also patrickholford. com. You can also teach yourself using the Psychocalisthenics DVD, available from www.pcals.com or www.HOLFORDirect.com. There is also a CD with music and prompts to follow once you have learned the exercises, a book that explains each exercise and a wall chart for quick reference.

© 1972, 2003, 2016 by Oscar Ichazo. Used with permission. All rights reserved. Psychocalisthenics® is a registered trademark of Oscar Ichazo in The United States of America. P-Cals® is a registered trademark of Oscar Ichazo in Canada.

Tests

Celiac test kits are available from leading pharmacies and online. YorkTest has a celiac test kit you can buy that measures IgATT, which is the specific antibody, the presence of which means you have celiac disease.

Their excellent service also includes an optional consultation with a BANT/CNHC-registered nutritional therapist, a guidebook and a food diary to help you work out what to avoid and what to eat instead.

Comprehensive Stool Test measures digestive markers and levels of both beneficial and pathogenic bacteria, as well as yeasts and parasites. This test is available via Biolab Medical Unit in London (www. biolab.co.uk), Genova Diagnostics (www.gdx.net) and Regenerus Labs (www.regeneruslabs.com) for Doctor's Data's MALDI-TOF test in the UK. These laboratories are referral laboratories, so testing can only be arranged via a doctor, a nutritional therapist or another registered healthcare professional. You can measure the activity of the enzyme beta-glucuronidase, which can generate carcinogens in the colon, with a stool test from Comprehensive Digestive Stool Analysis by Great Smokies Diagnostic Laboratories, which a clinical nutritionist can arrange for you.

Food Intolerance test. YorkTest Laboratories sells FoodScan, a convenient finger-prick mail-order service, with the added benefit of a clinical laboratory analysis. This is the only food intolerance test endorsed by Allergy UK. Designed as a simple two-step process, the First Step FoodScan is an indicator test that will generate a positive or negative result. If positive, your sample is then upgraded to the Second Step FoodScan 113 test, a comprehensive service that tests for 113 foods. The FoodScan 113 identifies the actual foods causing the intolerance and the level of intolerance. In addition, the service includes nutritionist consultations and comprehensive support and advice on managing your elimination diet. To order, call YorkTest Laboratories on 0800 130 0580 or visit www.yorktest.com.

Yoghurts My favourite yoghurts use *Lactobacillus acidophilus* and bifidobacteria. Look for those with labels stating, for example, 'BA yoghurt', or 'AB yoghurt', such as Longley Farm BA yoghurt.

Notes

Part I

1 Hardy, K., et al., 'The importance of dietary carbohydrate in human evolution' *Quarterly Review of Biology*, 2015;90(3):251–68.
2 Sipponen P., Hyvarinen H., Siurala M., '*H. pylori* corpus gastritis: Relation to acid output', *J Physiol Pharmacol*, 1996 Mar;47(1):151–9.
3 Slomianye, B.L., 'Gastric mucus viscosity and Heliobacter pylori', *Gut*, 1995 Oct;37(4):589–90.
4 Leoci, C., et al., 'Incidence and risk factors of duodenal ulcer. A retrospective cohort study', *J Clin Gastroenterol* 1995;20:104–9.

Part II

1 Fasano, A., 'Intestinal permeability and its regulation by zonulin: Diagnostic and therapeutic implications', *Clin Gastroenterol Hepatol*, 2012 Oct;10(10):1096–100.
2 Pfeiffer, C., original research paper (unpublished), Brain BioCenter. Pillay, D. et al., 'Zinc status in vitamin B6 deficiency', *Int J Vitam Nutr Res*, vol. 67 (1), pp 22–6 (1997).
3 Schlemmer U., et al., 'Phytate in foods and significance for humans: Food sources, intake, processing, bioavailability, protective role and analysis', *Mol Nutr Food*, res 2009;53:S330-75.
4 Ho K.S., et al., 'Stopping or reducing dietary fiber intake reduces constipation and its associated symptoms', *World J Gastroenterol*, 2012;18(33):4593–6.
5 Heizer, W.D., et al., 'The role of diet in symptoms of irritable bowel syndrome in adults: A narrative review', *J Am Diet Assoc*, 2009;109(7):1204–14.
6 Cockerell, K.M., 'Effects of linseeds on the symptoms of irritable bowel syndrome: A pilot randomised controlled trial', *J Hum Nutr Diet*, 2012 Oct;25(5):435–43.
7 Suares, N. and Ford, A., 'Systematic review: The effects of fibre in the management of chronic idiopathic constipation', *Aliment Pharmacol Ther*, 2011 Apr;33(8):895–901.
8 Chearskul, S., et al., 'Glycemic and lipid responses to glucomannan

in Thais with type-2 diabetes mellitus', *J Med Assoc Thai*, 2007 Oct;90(10):2150–7.

9 Yoshida, M., et al., 'Effect of plant sterols and glucomannan on lipids in individuals with and without type II diabetes', *Eur J Clin Nutr*, 2006 Apr;60(4):529–37; Chen, H.L., et al., 'Konjac supplement alleviated hypercholesterolemia and hyperglycemia in type-2 diabetic subjects: A randomized double-blind trial', *J Am Coll Nutr*, 2003 Feb;22(1):36–42.

10 Vuksan, V., et al., 'Beneficial effects of viscous dietary fiber from Konjac-mannan in subjects with the insulin resistance syndrome: Results of a controlled metabolic trial', *J Am Coll Nutr*, 2003 Feb;22(1):36–42; Vuksan, V., et al., 'Konjac-mannan (glucomannan) improves glycemia and other associated risk factors for coronary heart disease in type-2 diabetes. A randomized controlled metabolic trial', *Diabetes Care*, 1999 Jun;22(6):913–9.

11 Mito, A., data held in ION library, source unknown.

12 Walsh, D., unpublished study at GNC Research Center, Fargo, North Dakota (1982).

13 Holford, P., 'The effects of glucomannan on weight loss', Optimum Nutrition study report, 1984.

14 Zalewski, B.M., et al., 'The effect of glucomannan on body weight in overweight or obese children and adults: a systematic review of randomized controlled trials', *Nutrition*, 2015 Mar;31(3):437–42.

15 Chen, H.L., et al., 'Supplementation of konjac glucomannan into a low-fiber Chinese diet promoted bowel movement and improved colonic ecology in constipated adults: A placebo-controlled, diet-controlled trial', *J Am Coll Nutr*, 2008 Feb;27(1):102–8.

16 Lyon, M., Reichert, R., 'The effect of a novel viscous polysaccharide along with lifestyle changes on short-term weight loss and associated risk factor of overweight and obese adults', *Alternative Medicine Review*, 2010;115(1):68–75.

17 Brand-Miller, J., et al., 'Effects of PGX, a novel functional fibre, on acute and delayed postprandial glycaemia', *European Journal of Clinical Nutrition advance online publication*, 6 October 2010; doi:10.1038/ejcn.2010.199.

18 Jenkins, A.L., et al., 'Reduction of Postprandial Glycemia by the novel viscous polysaccharide PGX, in a dose-dependent manner, independent of food form', *J Am Coll of Nutr*, 2010;29(2):92–8.

19 Jenkins, A.L., 'Effect of adding the novel fiber, PGX®, to commonly consumed foods on glycemic response, glycemic index and GRIP: A simple and effective strategy for reducing post prandial blood glucose levels', *Nutr J*, 2010 Nov;22(9):58.

20 Lyon, M., and Kacinik, V., 'Is there a place for dietary fiber supplements in weight management?', *Curr Obes Rep*, 2012;1:59–67.

21 G.T. Macfarlane, et al., 'Bacterial metabolism and health-related effects of galacto-oligosaccharides and other prebiotics', *J Appl Microbiol.*, 2008 Feb;104(2):305–44.

22 Browne, H., et al., 'Culturing of "unculturable" human microbiota reveals novel taxa and extensive sporulation', *Nature*, 2016 533,p 543–6.

23 Mitsuuoka, T., 'Intestinal flora and aging', *Nutr Rev*, 1992;50(12):438–46.

24   Kadooka, Y., et al., 'Regulation of abdominal adiposity by probiotics (*Lactobacillus gasseri* SBT2055) in adults with obese tendencies in a randomized controlled trial', *European Journal of Clinical Nutrition*, June 2010.

25   Sanchez, M., et al, 'Effect of Lactobacillus rhamnosus CGMCC1.3724 supplementation on weight loss and maintenance in obese men and women', *Br J Nutr*, Apr 2014.

26   Madjd, A., et al., Comparison of the effect of daily consumption of probiotic compared with low-fat conventional yogurt on weight loss in healthy obese women following an energy-restricted diet: A randomized controlled trial', *Am J Clin Nutr*. 2016 Feb;103(2):323-9.

27   Karamali, M., et al., 'Effects of probiotic supplementation on glycaemic control and lipid profiles in gestational diabetes: A randomized, double-blind, placebo-controlled trial', *Diabetes Metab*, 2016 May 18. pii: S1262–3636(16)30401–3.

28   Woodard, G.A., et al., 'Probiotics improve outcomes after Roux-en-Y gastric bypass surgery: A prospective randomized trial', *J Gastrointest Surg*, 2009 Jul;13(7):1198–204.

29   Ohland, C.L., et al., 'Probiotic bacteria and intestinal epithelial barrier function', *American Journal of Physiology*, GI June 1, 2010 vol. 298.6.

30   See ref 26 above.

31   Guarner, F., et al., 'Consensus statements from the workshop "Probiotics and Health: Scientific Evidence"', *Nutricion Hospitalaria*, 2010;25(5):700–4.

32   Bernet, M.F., et al., 'Lactobacillus acidophilus LA1 binds to cultured human intestinal cell lines and inhibits cell attachment and cell invasion by enterovirulent bacteria', *Gut*, vol. 35, pp 483–9 (1994).

33   De Santis, S., et al., 'Nutritional Keys for Intestinal Barrier Modulation', *Front Immunol*, 2015 Dec 7;6:612.

34   Hill, M.J., 'Intestinal flora and endogenous vitamin synthesis', *European Journal of Cancer Prevention*, 1997, 6 Suppl 1:S43–5.

35   Borruel, N., et al., 'Increased mucosal TNF-a production in Crohn's disease can be down regulated ex vivo by probiotic bacteria', *Gut*, 2002;51:659–64.

36   Peltonen, R., et al., 'Changes of faecal flora in rheumatoid arthritis during fasting and one-year vegetarian diet', *Br J Rheumatol*, vol. 33, pp 638–43 (1994).

37   Majamaa, H. and Isolaui, E., 'Probiotics: A novel approach in the management of food allergy', *J Allergy Clin Immunol*, vol. 99, pp 179–85 (1997).

38   Hunter, J.O., 'Food allergy – or enterometabolic disorder?', *Lancet*, vol. 338, pp 495–6 (1991).

39   Cole, C.B. and Fuller, R., 'A note . . . on the coliform population of the neonatal rat gut', *J Appl Bacteriology*, vol. 56 (3), (1984).

40   M. Sanders, et al., 'An update on the use and investigation of probiotics in health and disease', *Gut*, 2013;62:787–96; Ritchie, Marina, L., and Romanuk, Tamara N., ' A meta-analysis of probiotic efficacy for gastrointestinal diseases', *PlosOne*, April 18, 2012; Goldenberg, J.Z.,

'Probiotics for the prevention of antibiotic-associated diarrhea in children', http://www.cochrane.org/CD004827, 2015

41 Goel, R.K. et al., 'Anti-ulcerogenic effect of banana powder (Musa sapientum var. paradisiaca) and its effect on mucosal resistance', *J Ethnopharmacol*, vol. 18 (1), pp 33–44 (1986).

42 see http://www.ncbi.nlm.nih.gov/pubmed/?term=kefir

43 Zamberi, N.R., et al., 'The antimetastatic and antiangiogenesis effects of kefir water on murine breast cancer cells', *Integr Cancer Ther*, 2016 May 26. pii: 1534735416642862.

44 Engen, P.A., et al, 'The gastrointestinal microbiome: Alcohol effects on the composition of intestinal microbiota', *Alcohol Res*, 2015;37(2):223–36. Review *Journal of the National Institute of Alcohol Abuse and Addiction* vol. 37, Number 2, 2015.

45 Madden, J.A., et al., 'Effect of probiotics on preventing disruption of the intestinal microflora following antibiotic therapy: A double-blind, placebo-controlled pilot study', *Int Immunopharmacol*, 2005;5(6):1091–7.

46 Cummings, J.H., et al., 'Prebiotic digestion and fermentation', *Am J Clin Nutr*, 2001;73(supp):415S–20S.

47 Vassallo, G., et al., 'Review article: Alcohol and gut microbiota – the possible role of gut microbiota modulation in the treatment of alcoholic liver disease', *Aliment Pharmacol Ther*, 2015 May;41(10):917–27.

48 Williams R. L. et al., 'Use of antibiotics in preventing recurrent acute otitis media and in treating otitis media with effusion, '*JAMA*. 1993 Sep 15;270(11):1344–51.

49 See the Center for Disease Dynamics, Economics & Policy's report on The State of the World's Antibiotics 2015 at https://cddep.org/sites/default/files/swa_2015_final.pdf

50 See http://www.independent.co.uk/life-style/health-and-families/health-news/373-thats-the-average-number-of-painkillers-we-each-take-in-a-year-is-it-too-many-516127.html

51 Bjarnason, I., et al., 'Intestinal permeability and inflammation in rheumatoid arthritis: Effects of non-steroidal anti-inflammatory drugs.' *Lancet*. 1984 Nov 24;2(8413):1171–4.

52 Ryan, A.J., et al., 'Gastrointestinal permeability following aspirin intake and prolonged running', *Med Sci Sports Exercise*, vol. 28 (6), pp 698–705 (1996).

53 Yap, .PR.,, Goh, K.L., 'Non-steroidal anti-inflammatory drugs (NSAIDs) induced dyspepsia', *Curr Pharm Des*, 2015;21(35):5073-81.

54 Allison, et al., 'Gastrointestinal damage associated with the use of nonsteroidal antiinflammatory drugs' *N Engl J Med*, vol. 327, pp 749–54 (1992)

55 Shin, Y.H., et al. 'The effect of capsaicin on salivary gland dysfunction', *Molecules*.,2016 Jun 25;21(7).

56 Catassi, R., et al., 'High prevalence of undiagnosed coeliac disease in 5280 Italian students screened by antigliadin antibodies', *Acta Paediatr*, vol. 84, pp 672–6 (1995).

57 Gerarduzzi,T., et al., *Journal of Pediatric Gastroenterology and Nutrition* 31 (suppl) 2000: S29, Abst. 104.

58 Screening for celiac disease in the general population and in high-risk

groups. Ludvigsson J. F. United European Gastroenterology Journal 2015, Vol. 3(2) 106–120

59   Gerarduzzi, T., et al., *Journal of Pediatric Gastroenterology and Nutrition* 31 (suppl) 2000: S29, Abst. 104.

60   ION research by Leonie Buswell (1996).

61   Carroccio, A., et al., 'Non-celiac wheat sensitivity diagnosed by double-blind placebo-controlled challenge: Exploring a new clinical entity', *Am J Gastroenterol*, 2012 Dec; 107(12):1898–906

62   Gao, X., '*High frequency of HMW-GS sequence variation through somatic hybridization between Agropyron elongatum and common wheat*', Planta, 2010, Jan;231(2):245–50.

63   van den Broeck, H., et al., 'Presence of celiac disease epitopes in modern and old hexaploid wheat varieties: Wheat breeding may have contributed to increased prevalence of celiac disease.'*Theor Appl Genet*, 2010 Nov; 121(8): 1527–39

64   Carnevali A. *et al.*, 'Role of Kamut® brand khorasan wheat in the counteraction of non-celiac wheat sensitivity and oxidative damage', *Food Res Int*, 2014, 63: 218–26

65   Valerii M.C., 'Responses of peripheral blood mononucleated cells from non-celiac gluten sensitive patients to various cereal sources', *Food Chem*, 2015 Jun 1;176:167–74

66   Zioudrou, C., et al., 'Opioid peptides derived from food proteins: The exorphins.', *J Biol Chem*, 1979, Apr 10;254(7): 2446–9.

67   Whittaker, A., et al., 'A khorasan wheat-based replacement diet improves risk profile of patients with type-2 diabetes mellitus (T2DM): A randomized crossover trial', *Eur J Nutr*, 2016, Feb 8; see also Whittaker, A., et al., 'An organic khorasan wheat-based replacement diet improves risk profile of patients with acute coronary syndrome: A randomized crossover trial', *Nutrients*, 2015 May 11;7(5):3401–15; see also Sofi, F., et al., 'Characterization of Khorasan wheat (Kamut) and impact of a replacement diet on cardiovascular risk factors: Cross-over dietary intervention study', *Eur J Clin Nutr*, 2013, Feb;67(2):190–5.

68   Sofi, F., et al., 'Effect of Triticum turgidum subsp. turanicum wheat on irritable bowel syndrome: A double-blinded randomised dietary intervention trial', *Br J Nutr*, 2014, Jun;111(1):1992–9

69   See a review of studies at https://www.patrickholford.com/advice/Kamut-khorasan-wheat-supergrain

70   Royal College of Physicians special report, 'Containing the Allergy Epidemic' (June 2003), Q *US News and World Report*, vol. 106(7), 77(2) (20 Feb. 1989).

71   Zhang, L., et al, 'Mast cells and irritable bowel syndrome: From the bench to the bedside', *Neurogastroenterol Motil*, 2016, 22:181–92.

72   Atkinson, W., et al., 'Food elimination based on IgG antibodies in irritable bowel syndrome: A randomised controlled trial', *Gut*, 2004;53:1459–64.; see also Zar, et al, 'Food-specific IgG4 antibody guided exclusion diet improves symptoms and rectal compliance in IBS', *Scand J Gastroenterol*', 2005, 40:800–807; see also Drisko, et al., 'Treating IBS with a food elimination diet, followed by food challenge and probiotics', *J Am Coll Nutr*, 2006, 25:514–22; see also Yang, C. and

Li, Y., 'The therapeutic effects of eliminating allergic foods according to food-specific IgG antibodies in irritable bowel syndrome', *Zhonghua Nei Ke Za Zhi*, 2007, 46:641–3; see also Guo, H., Jiang, T., Wang, J., 'The Value of Eliminating Foods According to Food-specific Immunoglobulin G Antibodies in Irritable Bowel Syndrome with Diarrhoea', *Journal of International Medical Research*, 2012; 40: 204–210.

73   Bentz, et al., 'Clinical relevance of IgG antibodies against food antigens in Crohn's disease: A double blind cross-over diet intervention study', *Digestion*, 2010, 81:252–64; see also 'Gunasekeera, et al., 'Treatment of Crohn's disease with an IgG4-guided exclusion diet: A randomised controlled trial', *Digestive Diseases and Sciences*, 2016, 61:1148–57.

74   Rees, T. et al., 'A prospective audit of food intolerance among migraine consumers in primary care clinical practice', *Headache Care* 2, 2005, 11–14; see also Alpay, K., et al., 'Diet restriction in migraine', based on IgG against foods: A clinical double-blind, randomised, cross-over trial', *Cephalagia*, 2010, 30, 829–37; see also Aydinlar, et al., 'IgG-based elimination diet in migraine plus IBS', *Headache*, 2013, 53:514–25

75   Lewis, J. et al., 'Eliminating immunologically-reactive foods from the diet and its effect on body composition and quality of life in overweight persons', *Journal of Obesity & Weight loss Therapy*, 2012, 2:1.

76   Hardman, G. and Hart, G., 'Dietary advice based on food specific IgG results', *Nutrition and Food Science*, 2007, 37:16–23 plus further analysis of data provided by the author.

77   Margioris, A.N., 'Fatty acids and postprandial inflammation', *Current Opinion in Clinical Nutrition & Metabolic Care,* 2009; 12(2):129–37.

78   Benton D. et al., 'Impact of consuming a milk drink containing a probiotic on mood and cognition', *European Journal of Clinical Nutrition*, 2007; 61 (3):355–61.

79   Randolph, T., 'Allergy as a causative factor of fatigue, irritability and behaviour problems of children', *Journal of Paediatrics*, 1947; 31:560; Rowe, A., 'Allergic toxemia and fatigue', *Annals of Allergy,* 1959;17: 9; Speer, G., 'Allergy of the Nervous System', *Thomas,* 1970; Campbell, M., 'Neurologic manifestations of allergic disease', *Annals of Allergy*, 1973; 31:485; Hall, K., 'Allergy of the nervous system: A review', *Annals of Allergy,* 1976; 36: 49–64; Pippere, V., 'Some varieties of food intolerance in psychiatric patients' *Nutrition and Health,* 1984; 3:125–36; Pfeiffer, C., and Holford, P., *Mental Illness and Schizophrenia: The Nutrition Connection*, 1989, Thorsons; Tuormaa, T., *An Alternative to Psychiatry,* 1991, The Book Guild; Parker, G. and Watkins, T., 'Treatment-resistant depression: When antidepressant drug intolerance may indicate food intolerance', *Australian and New Zealand Journal of Psychiatry.*2002 Apr;36(2):263–5.

80   Egger, J., et al., 'Controlled trial of oligoantigenic diet treatment in the hyperkinetic syndrome', *Lancet*, 1985; 1: 540–5.

81   Feingold, B., 'Dietary management of behaviour and learning disabilities', *Nutrition and Behaviour*, 1981: 37, S.A. Miller (ed), Franklin Institute Press.

82   Ciacci, C., et al., 'Depressive symptoms in adult celiac disease', *Scandinavian journal of gastroenterology*, 1998 Mar;33(3):247–50.

83   Ford, R.P., 'The gluten syndrome: A neurological disease', *Medical Hypotheses,* 2009 Sep;73(3):438–40.

84   Roos, C., et al., 'A discriminating messenger RNA signature for bipolar disorder formed by an aberrant expression of inflammatory genes in monocytes', *Archives of General Psychiatry,* 2008;65(4):395–407; also see S. Zeugmann, et al., 'Inflammatory biomarkers in 70 depressed inpatients with and without the metabolic syndrome.' *Journal of Clinical Psychiatry,* 2010 Feb 9; also see B. Fang, et al., 'Disturbed sleep: Linking allergic rhinitis, mood and suicidal behavior', *Frontiers of Bioscience* (Schol Ed), 2010 Jan 1;2:30–46.

85   Holford, P., et al., The 100% Health Survey, p.11–12, www. patrickholford.com

86   Vogelzangs, N., et al., 'Urinary cortisol and six-year risk of all-cause and cardiovascular mortality', *Journal of Clinical Endocrinology and Metabolism,* (2010), vol. 95(11), pp. 4959–64.

87   Kivmaki M. et al., 'Common mental disorder and obesity: Insight from four repeat measures over 19 years: Prospective Whitehall II cohort study', *British Medical Journal,* 2009, vol. 339:b3765 (available online at http://www.bmj.com/content/339/bmj.b3765.full). ; also see Johansson, L., et al., 'Midlife psychological stress and risk of dementia: A 35-year longitudinal population study', *Brain,* 2010, vol. 133, pp. 2217–24.; also see Eriksson, A.K., et al., 'Psychological distress and risk of pre-diabetes and type-2 diabetes in a prospective study of Swedish middle-aged men and women', *Diabetic Medicine,* 2008, vol. 25, pp. 834–42.

88   Aboa-Eboule, C., et al., 'Job strain and risk of acute recurrent coronary heart disease events', *Journal of the American Medical Association,* 2007, vol. 298(14), pp. 1652–60.

89   Mind, 'Mental Health at Work: Populus Survey of Workers in England and Wales', 2013.

90   Barreau, F., et al., 'Neonatal maternal deprivation triggers long term alterations in colonic epithelial barrier and mucosal immunity in rats', *Gut,* 2004 April; 53(4): 501–506.

91 · Gareau, M.G., et al., 'Probiotic treatment of rat pups normalises corticosterone release and ameliorates colonic dysfunction induced by maternal separation', *Gut,* 2007; 56:1522–8.

Part III

1   Drossman, D.A., et al., 'US house-holder survey of functional Gl disorders: Prevalence, sociodemography and health impact', *Dig Dis Sci,* vol. 38, pp 1569–80 (1993).

2   Harris, G. and Koli E., 'Lucrative drug, danger signals and the FDA', *New York Times,* 10 June 2005 .

3   Shoshana, J., et al., 'Acid-suppressive medication use and the risk for nosocomial gastrointestinal tract bleeding', *Archives of Internal Medicine,* 2011;171(11):991–7.

4   Editorial: Overprescribing proton pump inhibitors, *British Medical Journal,* 2008, vol. 336, pp 2–3.

5   Gomm W et al., 'Association of Proton Pump Inhibitors With Risk of

Dementia: A Pharmacoepidemiological Claims Data Analysis', J AMA Neurol. 2016 Apr 1;73(4):410-6

6   Lam, J.R., et al., 'Proton pump inhibitor and histamine 2 receptor antagonist use and vitamin B12 deficiency', *JAMA*, 2013, Dec 11;310(22):2435–42.

7   Andrès E., et al., 'Vitamin B_{12} (cobalamin) deficiency in elderly patients', *CMAJ*, August 2004;171(3):251–9

8   Yang, Y.X., et al., 'Long-term proton pump inhibitor therapy and risk of hip fracture', *Journal of the American Medical Association*, 2006 Dec 27;296(24):2947–53.

9   Cunningham, R., 'Is over-use of proton pump inhibitors fuelling the current epidemic of Clostridium difficile-associated diarrhoea?', *Journal of Hospital Infection*, 2008, vol. 70 (1), pp 1–6.

10 Lambert, A.A., et al., 'Risk of community-acquired pneumonia with outpatient proton-pump inhibitor therapy: A systematic review and meta-analysis', PLoS One. 2015 Jun 4;10(6):e0128004.

11 See http://www.independent.co.uk/life-style/health-and-families/health-news/373-thats-the-average-number-of-painkillers-we-each-take-in-a-year-is-it-too-many-516127.html

12 Graham, D.Y. and Opekun, A.R., et al, 'Visible small-intestinal mucosal injury in chronic NSAID users', *Clinical Gastroenterology and Hepatology*, 2005, vol. 3(1), pp 55–9.

13 Press release: 'Study shows long-term use of NSAIDs causes severe intestinal damage', *American Gastroenterological Association*, 3 January 2005.

14 Press release issued by *Annual Digestive Disease Week*, 16 May 2005, referring to a study later published as Goldstein, J.L., Johanson, J.F., et al., 'Healing of gastric ulcers with esomeprazole versus ranitidine in patients who continued to receive NSAID therapy: A randomized trial', *American Journal of Gastroenterology*, 2005, vol. 100(12), pp 2650–7.

15 Jan Magnus Bjordal, N., et al., 'Non-steroidal anti-inflammatory drugs, including cyclo-oxygenase-2 inhibitors, in osteoarthritic knee pain: Meta-analysis of randomised placebo controlled trials', *British Medical Journal*, 2004, vol. 329, pp 1317

16 See http://davidhealy.org/humira-in-ulcerative-colitis/

17 Tulstrup, M.V., et al., 'Antibiotic treatment affects intestinal permeability and gut microbial composition in Wistar rats dependent on antibiotic class', *PLoS One*, 2015 Dec 21;10(12):e0144854.

18 See http://www.dailymail.co.uk/health/article-3593515/Antibiotics-got-rid-chest-infection-Jane-says-destroyed-health.html.

19 Quigley, M., and Abu-Shanab, A., 'Small intestinal bacterial overgrowth', *Infect Dis Clin North Am*, 2010, Dec;24(4):943–59, viii-ix.

20 Menees, S.B., et al., 'The efficacy and safety of rifaximin for the irritable bowel syndrome: A systematic review and meta-analysis',

21 100% Health Survey, Holford & Associates, January 2011

22 Galland, L., 'Leaky gut syndrome: Breaking the vicious cycle', *Townsend Letter for Doctors*, Aug/Sept 1995.

23 Hollon, J., et al., 'Effect of gliadin on permeability of intestinal biopsy explants from celiac disease patients and patients with non-celiac gluten

sensitivity', *Nutrients*, 2015 Feb 27;7(3):1565–76.

24 Northrop-Clewes, C.A., and Downes, R.M., 'Chronic diarrhoea and malnutrition in the Gambia: Studies on intestinal permeability', *Trans R Soc Trop Med Hyg*, vol. 85 (1), pp 8–11 (1991).

25 Sudduth, W.H., 'The role of bacteria and enterotoxemia in physical addition to alcohol', *Microecology and Therapy*, vol. 18 (1989).

26 Bernard, et al., 'Increased intestinal permeability in bronchial asthma', *Allergy Clin Immunol*, vol. 97, pp 1173–8 (1996).

27 Andre, C., et al., 'Measurement of intestinal permeability to mannitol and lactulose as a means of diagnosing food allergy and evaluating therapeutic effectiveness of disodium cromoglycate', *Ann Allergy*, 1987 Nov;59(5 Pt 2):127–30.

28 Healy, D., 'Humira in ulcerative colitis', 2013, Jul 29 see also; van der Hulst, R.R., 'Glutamine and the preservation of gut integrity', *Lancet*, vol. 341, Issue 8857, Pages 1363–5.

29 De Santis, S., et al., 'Nutritional keys for intestinal barrier modulation', *Front Immunol*, 2015 Dec 7;6:612.

30 Kong, J., et al., 'Novel role of the vitamin D receptor in maintaining the integrity of the intestinal mucosal barrier', *Am J Physiol Gastrointest Liver Physiol*, 2008, Jan;294(1):G208–16. Epub 2007 Oct 25.

31 Ranjit, N., et al., 'Psychosocial factors and inflammation in the multi-ethnic study of atherosclerosis', *Archives of Internal Medicine*, 2007;167:174–81.

32 Masood, A., et al., 'Serum high sensitivity C-reactive protein levels and the severity of coronary atherosclerosis assessed by angiographic gensini score', *Journal of the Pakistan Medical Association*, 2011 Apr;61(4):325–7.

33 Di Napoli, M., et al., 'C-reactive protein level measurement improves mortality prediction when added to the spontaneous intracerebral hemorrhage score', *Stroke*, 2011, May;42(5):1230–6. Epub 2011 Apr 7.

34 Hänninen, O., et al., 'Antioxidants in vegan diet and rheumatic disorders', *Toxicology*, 2000, vol. 155 (1–3), pp 45–53.

35 Beauchamp, G., et al., 'Ibuprofen-like activity in extra-virgin olive oil', *Nature*, 2005, vol. 437, pp 45–46.

36 Jagetia, G.C. and Aggarwal, B.B., 'Spicing up of the immune system by curcumin', *Journal of Clinical Immunology*, 2007, vol. 27 (1), pp 19–35.

37 Lemay, M., et al, 'In vitro and ex vivo cyclooxygenase inhibition by a hops extract', *Asia Pacific Journal of Clinical Nutrition*, 2004, vol. 13 (suppl), pp S110.

38 K.Y. Wang, et al., 'Effects of ingesting Lactobacillus- and Bifidobacterium containing yogurt in subjects with colonised Helicobacter pylori', *American Journal of Clinical Nutrition*, Sept 2004; 80(3):737–41.

39 Parascho, S., et al., 'In vitro and in vivo activities of chios mastic gum extracts and constituents against helicobacter pylori, antimicrobial agents and chemotherapy', *Antimicrobial Agents and Chemotherapy*, 2007;51(2):551–9.

40 Xing, J., et al., 'Effects of sea buckthorn (Hippopha. rhamnoides L.) seed and pulp oils on experimental models of gastric ulcer in rats', *Fitoterapia*, Dec 2002;73(7–8):644–50.

41   Pearson, A., et al., 'Intestinal permeability in children with Crohn's
     disease and celiac disease', *BMJ*, vol. 285, p. 20 (1982).
42   Sanderson, I.R., et al., 'Improvement of abnormal lactulose/rhamnose
     permeability in active Crohn's disease of the small bowel by an
     elemental diet', *Gut*, vol. 28, pp 1073–6 (1987).
43   Hlavaty, T., et al., 'Vitamin D therapy in inflammatory bowel diseases:
     Who, in what form, and how much?', *J Crohns Colitis*, 2015 Feb;9(2):198–
     209. Review.
44   Maagaard L. et al., 'Follow-up of patients with functional bowel
     symptoms treated with a low FODMAP diet', *World J Gastroenterol*, 2016
     Apr 21;22(15):4009–19
45   Gerarduzzi, T., et al., *Journal of Pediatric Gastroenterology and Nutrition*
     31 (suppl) 2000: S29, Abst. 104.
46   I. Dahlbom, et al., 'Prediction of clinical and mucosal severity of coeliac
     disease and dermatitis herpetiformis by quantification of IgA/IgG serum
     antibodies to tissue transglutaminase', *J Pediatr Gastroenterol Nutr*, 2010
     Feb;50(2):140–6.
47   Cascella, N.G.,'Prevalence of celiac disease and gluten sensitivity in the
     United States clinical antipsychotic trials of intervention effectiveness
     study population', *Schizophr Bull.* 2011 Jan;37(1):94–100.
48   Ibid.
49   Mora, S., et al., 'Reversal of low bone density with a gluten-free diet
     in children and adolescents with celiac disease', *Am J Clin Nutr*, 1998
     Mar;67(3):477–81.
50   Hoggan, R., 'Considering wheat, rye, and barley proteins as aids to
     carcinogens', *Med Hypotheses*, 1997, vol. 49, pp. 285–288
51   Mendez, E., (2006), 'Confirmation of the cereal type in oat products
     highly contaminated with gluten', *Journal of the American Dietetic
     Association*, 106 (5); see also Ciclitira P.J., Ellis H.J., Lundin K.E.A.
     (2005) 'Gluten-free diet – what is toxic?', *Best Practice and Research
     Clinical Gastroenterology*, 2005, 19 (3): 359 – 371.
52   Janatuinen, E.K, et al., (2002). 'No harm from five year ingestion
     of oats in coeliac disease', *Gut*, 2002, 50: 332 – 335; see also
     Kemppainen, T.A., et al., et al., 'Unkilned and large amounts of
     oats in the coeliac disease diet: a randomized,controlled study',
     2008;43(9):1094 101.
53   Lundin K. et al., Oats induced villous atrophy in coeliac disease, *Gut*,
     2003, 52:1649–1652
54   See http://news.bbc.co.uk/1/hi/health/669401.stm
55   Thorne, G.M., 'Diagnosis of infectious diarrheal diseases', *Infect Dis Clin
     North Am*, 1988, 2(3):747–51
56   Wheeler, J.G. et al., 'Study of infectious intestinal disease in England:
     Rates in the community, presenting to general practice, and reported to
     national surveillance. The Infectious Intestinal Disease Study Executive',
     BMJ, 1999 Apr 17;318(7190):1046–50
57   Wolfe, M.S., *Clin Microbiology Review*, vol 5 (1), pp 93–100 (1992)
58   Eastham, E.J. et al., 'Diagnosis of *Giardia lamblia* infection as a cause of
     diarrhoea', *Lancet*, pp 950–51 (1976).
59   Bueno, Hermann, *Uninvited Guests*, Keats (1996).

60 Dogruman-Al F et al., 'Comparison of methods for detection of Blastocystis infection in routinely submitted stool samples, and also in IBS/IBD Patients in Ankara, Turkey.' PLoS One, 2010 Nov 18;5(11):e15484

61 See http://dailymail.co.uk/health/article-2520986/You-catch-giardia-drinking-British-water-foregin-parasite-giardia-lamblia.html

62 Wynburn-Mason, R. The Causation of Rheumatoid Disease and Many Human Cancers: a new Concept in Medicine, Iji publishing Company, Tokyo, (1978)

63 Russo, A.R., et al., 'Presumptive evidence for Blastocystis hominis as a cause of colitis', Arch Intern Med, vol.148 (5), p 1064 (1988). Hussain Quadri, S.M., Al-Okaili, G.A. and Al-Dayel, F., 'Clinical significance of Blastocystis hominis', J Clin Microbiol, vol .27 (11), pp 2407–9 (1989). Kain, K.C., et al., 'Epidemiology and clinical features associated with Blastocystis hominis infection', Diagn Microbiol Infect Dis, vol. 8 (4), pp 234–44 (1987).

64 See reference 2 above.

65 Elgayyar, M., et al., 'Antimicrobial activity of essential oils from plants against selected pathogenic and saprophytic microorganisms', J Food Prot, 2001 Jul;64(7):1019–24

66 Kyme, P. et al., 'C/EBPε mediates nicotinamide-enhanced clearance of Staphylococcus aureus in mice.' J Clin Invest, 2012 Sep 4;122(9):3316–29

67 Yinghjian, Z. and Liangyou, R., 'Leptin signaling and leptin resistance', Front Med, Jun 2013, vol. 7, issue 2, 207–222.

68 Lewis, J., et al., 'Eliminating immunologically-reactive foods from the diet and its effect on body composition and quality of life in overweight persons', J Obes Weig Los Ther, 2012, 2:1

69 Buhner, S., et al., 'Activation of human enteric neurons by supernatants of colonic biopsy specimens from patients with irritable bowel syndrome', Gastroenterology, 2009;137(4):1425–34

70 Sameer, Z., et al, 'Food-specific serum IgG4 and IgE titers to common food antigens in irritable bowel syndrome', American Journal of Gastroenterology, 2005; 100:p1550–7

71 Biesiekierski, J.R., et al.,'Gluten causes gastrointestinal symptoms in subjects without celiac disease: A double-blind randomized placebo-controlled trial', Am J Gastroenterol, 2011 Mar;106(3):508–14

72 Jellema, P., 'Lactose malabsorption and intolerance: A systematic review on the diagnostic value of gastrointestinal symptoms and self-reported milk intolerance', QJM, 2010 Aug;103(8):555–72.

73 Atkinson, W., et al., 'Food elimination based on IgG antibodies in irritable bowel syndrome: A randomised controlled trial', Gut, 2004;53:1459–64

74 Lillestøl, K., et al., 'Anxiety and depression in patients with self-reported food hypersensitivity', General Hospital Psychiatry, 2010 Jan-Feb; 32(1):42–8

75 Moayyedi, P., et al., 'The efficacy of probiotics in the treatment of irritable bowel syndrome: A systematic review', Gut, 2010;59(3):325–32

76 Silk, D.B., et al., 'Clinical trial: The effects of a trans-galactooligosaccharide prebiotic on faecal microbiota and symptoms

in irritable bowel syndrome', *Aliment Pharmacology and Therapeutics*, 2009;29(5):508–18

77 Jalanka-Tuovinen, J., et al., 'Intestinal microbiota in healthy adults: Temporal analysis reveals individual and common core and relation to intestinal symptoms, *PLos One*, 2011,;6(7);e23035

78 Pimentel, M., et al, 'Normalisation of lactulose breath testing bowel syndrome: A double blind, randomized, placebo-controlled study', *Am J Gastroenterol*, 2003, Feb;98(2):412–9.

79 Pyleris, E., et al., 'The prevalence of overgrowth by aerobic bacteria in the small intestine by small bowel culture: Relationship with irritable bowel syndrome', *Dig Dis Sci*, 2012, May;57(5): 1321–9 Epub 2012 Jan 20.

80 Lin, H.C., 'Small intestinal bacterial overgrowth: A framework for understanding irritable bowel syndrome', *Jama*, 2004, Aug 18;292(7):852–8

81 Compare, D., 'Effects of long-term PPI treatment on producing bowel symptoms and SIBO', *Eur J Clin Invest*, 2011, Apr;41(4):380–6

82 Maagaard, L. et al., 'Follow-up of patients with functional bowel symptoms treated with a low FODMAP diet', *World J Gastroentero*, 2016 Apr 21;22(15):4009–19

83 Chen, C. and Tao, C., 'A randomized clinical trial of berberine hydrochloride in patients with diarrhea-predominant irritable bowel syndrome', *Phytother Res*, 2015 Nov;29(11):1822–7. doi: 10.1002/ ptr.5475. Epub 2015 Sep 24.

84 Grigoleit, H.G. and Grigoleit, P., 'Gastrointestinal clinical pharmacology of peppermint oil, *Phytomedicine*, 2005, Aug;12(8):607–11.

85 Grigoleit H.G. and Grigoleit P., 'Pharmacology and preclinical pharmacokinetics of peppermint oil', *Phytomedicine*, 2005, Aug;12(8):612–6 see also; Kingham, J.G., 'Peppermint oil and colon spasm', *Lancet*, 1995, 346.8981.

86 Braun, L. and Cohen, M., 'Herbs and natural supplements: An evidence based guide 3rd edition, *Churchill Livingstone*, 2010 see also; Logan, A.C. and Beaulne, T.M., 'The treatment of small intestinal bacterial overgrowth with enteric-coated peppermint oil: A case report', *Altern Med Rev*, 2002, Oct;7(5):410–7.

87 Gwee KA, et al., 'Psychometric scores and persistence of irritable bowel after infectious diarrhoea', Lancet. 1996 Jan 20;347(8995):150-3.

88 Adam, J., et al., 'Controlled double blind clinical trials of Saccharomyces boulardii': Multi centre study involving 25 physicians and 388 cases', *Medicine et Chirugie Digestives* 1976; 5:401–05

89 Sasaki, H., et al., 'Innovative preparation of curcumin for improved oral bioavailability', Biol Pharm Bull, 2011;34(5):660–5.

90 Rigden, S., et al., 'Management of chronic fatigue symptoms by tailored nutritional intervention using a program designed to support hepatic detoxification', *HealthComm Inc*

91 Rigden, S., et al., 'Evaluation of the effect of a modified entero-hepatic resuscitation program in chronic fatigue syndrome patients', *Functional Medicine Research Center*, 1997.

92 Myhill, S., et al., 'Targeting mitochondrial dysfunction in the treatment of Myalgic Encephalomyelitis/Chronic Fatigue Syndrome (ME/CFS): A

clinical audit', *International Journal of Clinical Experimental Medicine*, 2013;6(1):1–15

93 Vassallo, G., et al, Review article: 'Alcohol and gut microbiota: The possible role of gut microbiota modulation in the treatment of alcoholic liver disease', *Aliment Pharmacol Ther*, 2015, May;41(10):917–27.

94 Trinkley, K.E., et al., 'Prescribing patterns for outpatient treatment of constipation, irritable bowel syndrome-related constipation, and opioid-induced constipation: A retrospective cross-sectional study', *J Manag Care Spec Pharm*, 2015 Nov;21(11):1077–87.

95 Jacobs, E.J. and White, E., 'Constipation, laxative use and colon cancer among middle-aged adults', *Epidemiology*, vol. 9 (4), pp 385–91 (1998).

96 Eskesen, D. and Jespersen, L.,'Effect of the probiotic strain *Bifidobacterium animalis* subsp. lactis, BB-12®, on defecation frequency in healthy subjects with low defecation frequency and abdominal discomfort: A randomised, double-blind, placebo-controlled, parallel-group trial', *Br J Nutr*, 2015 Nov 28;114(10):1638–46. doi: 10.1017/S0007114515003347. Epub 2015 Sep 18.

97 Naylor, G.M., et al., 'Why does Japan have a high incidence of gastric cancer? Comparison of gastritis between UK and Japanese patients', *Gut*, 2006, Nov;55(11): 1545–52

98 Bailey, C.E., et al., 'Increasing disparities in the age-related incidences of colon and rectal cancers in the United States, 1975–2010', JAMA Surg, 2015, Jan;150(1):17–22

99 Donaldson, M.S., 'Nutrition and cancer: A review of the evidence for an anti-cancer diet', 2004 Oct 20;3:19

100 Abid, Z. et al., 'Meat, dairy, and cancer', *Am J Clin Nutr*, 2014 Jul;100 Suppl 1:386S-93S. doi: 10.3945/ajcn.113.071597. Epub 2014 May 21.

101 Reddy, S., et al., 'Faecal pH, bile acid and sterol concentrations in premenopausal Indian and white vegetarian compared with white omnivores', *Br J Nutr*, vol. 79, pp 495–500 (1998).

102 Hambly, R.J., et al., 'Effects of high- and low-risk diets on gut microflora-associated biomarkers of colon cancer in human flora associated rats', *Nutr Cancer*, vol. 27 (3), pp 250–5 (1997).

103 Nijhoff, W.A., et al., 'Effects of consumption of Brussels sprouts on intestinal and lymphocytic glutathione S-transferases in humans' *Carcinogenesis*. 1995 Sep;16(9):2125–8

Index

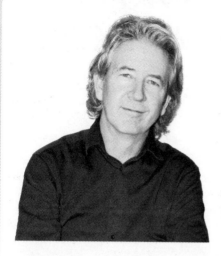

patrick HOLFORD
100% HEALTH WORKSHOPS

TOTAL HEALTH TRANSFORMATION

Avoid the mid-life health meltdown. Beat the bulge. Give your body a total transformation. Find out how to radically improve your health in this highly informative and motivating workshop. You leave with your own personalised health plan and the tools to be successful.

OPTIMUM EXERCISE IN 15 MINUTES

How do you keep fit, strong, supple and full of energy? The habit of exercise can be hard to keep up, but how much easier would it be if all you needed was 15 minutes every day? This workshop shows you four simple ways to achieve these goals in 15 minutes a day.

OPTIMUM NUTRITION FOR THE MIND

There is no need to have declining energy, memory, motivation and mood. In this one-day workshop you will learn everything Patrick's learnt in 35 years exploring nutrition for mental health.

THE POWER OF CONNECTION

Is life an adventure or an ordeal? Are you having a good time, full of 'joie de vivre' or are you bored or in discomfort of one sort or another, be it emotional or mental anguish, stress or physical pain? Does life make sense or do you have the feeling there's another level of existence but don't know how to get there? Patrick Holford shares deepest wisdoms that help you feel fully alive and awake and connected on all levels, living a purposeful life.

For latest seminars and workshops visit
www.patrickholford.com/events